Drugging For "Health"

Why the Paradigm Must Change

Kenneth C. Dyer, Jr.

Disclaimer: I am not a medical doctor. I have not been misinformed, indoctrinated and/or brainwashed into the paradigm of toxic drugs for so-called "health". For the most part, I do not condone the nonsense that is called "medical care" in this country and abroad. I **do have** training in medicinal herbalism and nutritional medicine, but I **do not** have the legal right to diagnose illness or prescribe treatments. I do not assume liability for the misuse of any information contained herein. The information contained within this book is offered to provide you with **education only** on beneficial concepts regarding your health and well-being in an effort to inform you of what your real options are regarding your healthcare. Every patient has different problems and requires different care plans, therefore please consult your primary care physician before beginning any new program, keeping in mind that the most beneficial kind of primary care physician is one who practices holistic, naturopathic techniques and only uses drugs as a last resort.

ISBN-13:
978-1508544371

ISBN-10:
1508544379

The drug companies in collusion with the FDA, Federal Government, American Medical Association, American Cancer Society, American Diabetes Association, et al, have created a ruthless monopoly on the medical system. They are suppressing **natural cures** for cancer, MRSA and more. They're inventing fake "scientific" studies and perpetuating myths such as "HIV Causes AIDS" and "Cholesterol Causes Heart Disease", inventing phony disorders such as "ADHD", pushing deadly toxic vaccines and lying about their safety and efficacy + much, much more, all in an effort to maintain their control, push more drugs, increase their sales and maximize profits. The truth is that they are killing millions of people per year under the guise of "healing" people with *unnecessary* drugs, surgeries and so-called "treatments".

Virtually all health concerns are manageable through diet, nutrition and natural supplements, **including cancer**. This book will provide you with key information needed to become your own doctor and escape the brutal and inhumane medical monopoly where profits come first and the health of the people comes last. This book will show you how to reclaim your power and your health. This book represents the new paradigm of nutrition, **not drugs**, for health.

"One of the great myths about natural medicines is that they are not scientific. The fact of the matter is that for most common illnesses there is greater support in the medical literature for a natural approach than there is for drugs or surgery."

- Dr. Michael Murray, N.D.

"Drugs never cure disease. They merely hush the voice of nature's protest, and pull down the danger signals she erects along the pathway of transgression. Any poison taken into the system has to be reckoned with later on even though it palliates present symptoms. Pain may disappear, but the patient is left in worse condition, though unconscious of it at the time."

- Dr. Daniel H. Kress, M.D.

"I haven't been to a doctor for aeons because I prefer to be healed than be made still sicker."

- David Icke

"The genius suggestion that you'll be healthier if you fill your body with toxic drugs is exactly the same as saying that filling a helium balloon with lead will make it float better! There is simply no place for toxins in a healthy body. Period."

- Author

The original version of the Hippocratic Oath:

I swear by Apollo the physician, and Aesculapius the surgeon, likewise Hygeia and Panacea, and call all the gods and goddesses to witness, that I will observe and keep this underwritten oath, to the utmost of my power and judgment.

I will reverence my master who taught me the art. Equally with my parents, will I allow him things necessary for his support, and will consider his sons as brothers. I will teach them my art without reward or agreement; and I will impart all my acquirement, instructions, and whatever I know, to my master's children, as to my own; and likewise to all my pupils, who shall bind and tie themselves by a professional oath, but to none else.

With regard to healing the sick, I will devise and order for them the best diet, according to my judgment and means; and I will take care that they suffer no hurt or damage.

Nor shall any man's entreaty prevail upon me to administer poison to anyone; neither will I counsel any man to do so. Moreover, I will give no sort of medicine to any pregnant woman, with a view to destroy the child.

Further, I will comport myself and use my knowledge in a godly manner.

I will not cut for the stone, but will commit that affair entirely to the surgeons.

Whatsoever house I may enter, my visit shall be for the convenience and advantage of the patient; and I will willingly refrain from doing any injury or wrong from falsehood, and (in an especial manner) from acts of an amorous nature, whatever may be the rank of those who it may be my duty to cure, whether mistress or servant, bond or free.

Whatever, in the course of my practice, I may see or hear (even when not invited), whatever I may happen to obtain knowledge of, if it be not proper to repeat it, I will keep sacred and secret within my own breast.

If I faithfully observe this oath, may I thrive and prosper in my fortune and profession, and live in the estimation of posterity; or on breach thereof, may the reverse be my fate!

CONTENTS

Preface to Second Edition

The first edition of this book came out a little over one year ago. Since then I've been continuing my self-education as well as my diet plan and nutritional supplement regimen consisting of multi-vitamins, minerals, amino acids, herbs, and other natural substances. I taylor made my own supplement regimen with the help of Dr. Robert Atkins, may he R.I.P. If I have an official doctor it's *myself*, of course, with the help of my books and resources, but Dr. Atkins is special to me. His advice has made a huge difference in my life! His book *Dr. Atkins' Vita-Nutrient Solution: Nature's Answer to Drugs* was my personal guide in Nov. 2014 when I started my plan. His book outlines all the best supplements to take according to what health problems plague you, and he gives detailed dosage information and lots of other information concerning each supplement, and yes, it does include information on several common medicinal herbs as well.

My nutraceutical plan has been lowered in quantity since I first began. As my conditions have stabilized I have decreased the dosages on my natural medicines, for example, at one point I was on a ten-herb blend, an herbal tincture that I produced myself for the purpose of lowering my blood pressure. I took that batch until it was gone and then I discontinued it. I made a point to check my blood pressure over the next week or so after I stopped taking it, and my blood pressure remains stable without it. At last reading my blood pressure was a mere 121/71 which is incredible for me!

My weight has continued to drop since I've started. I've remained failthful to the diet plan that I so very firmly believe in, the low carb diet made famous by my doctor, Dr. Atkins and my overall health has improved dramatically. I am very aware that there is no "one size fits all" diet plan, for example some people can't tolerate too much protein in their diets, some people have allergies and food sensitivities and so forth and so on, but generally speaking, when it comes to people who only have "normal" health issues who can tolerate protein, etc., there is simply no better or healthier diet plan and that's because it almost completely removes the poison called sugar from your diet and when that happens health improves almost immediately. I do address the diet throughout the text of this entire book making point after point after point about the benefits of low carb diets (including that it protects against cancer) and provide scientific data in the Appendix as well. Many of the myths concerning low carb diets, for example the one that says that "low carb diets raise cholesterol and cause heart attacks", are quite thoroughly debunked in the text of this book as well. I am living proof of the diet's effectiveness, not only for losing weight, but for overall general health.

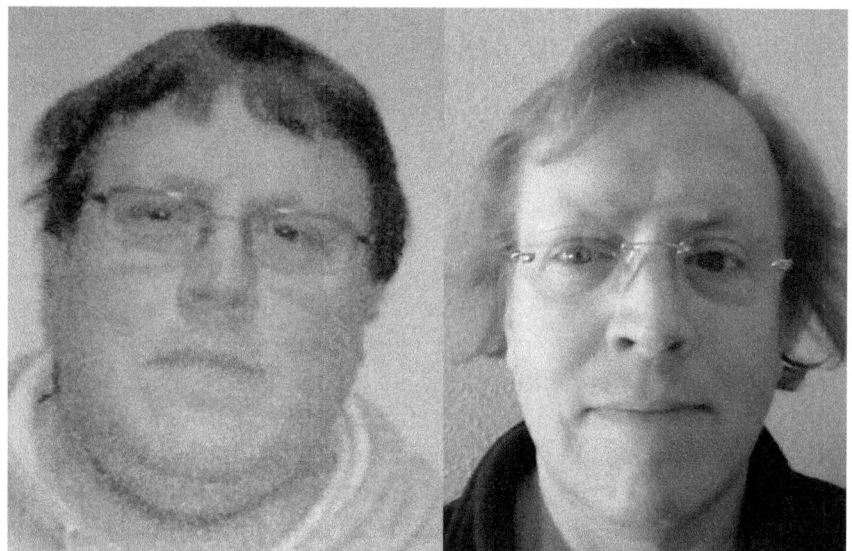

December of 2011 and July of 2016.

My weight was over 300 lbs when I started this plan, my blood pressure was high, I had blood sugar readings in the 500s, I was tired all the time, my gout was acting up and at one point I was almost bedridden because of it and had to use crutches to get around for a few days. So, in a nutshell, I was in shit health and I felt like shit too. I had been studying natural medicine for years, but had recently done an extensive crash course in self-study as well as earning certificates in herbal medicine and nutrition from courses that I found online. I've now been very, very seriously studying natural medicines for about two years, and before that I had been casually studying for about six years. Overall, despite not having an "official diploma" hanging on my wall, I would say that I am very knowledgeable in the area of natural medicine. I'm no expert, but I'm by no means a novice. I trust my skill sets to take care of myself for the rest of my life, and I'd say that's a pretty good thing for me to have, knowledge of self-administering natural medicines.

My weight has since dropped to 219 and still dropping, and that's because I don't eat sugar or foods that turn into sugar. Despite being diagnosed a type 2 diabetic my blood sugar is absolutely stabilized and consistently reads in the normal range of 70-120 or so, and that's because I don't eat sugar or foods that turn into sugar. My cholesterol consistently reads in the normal range, as do my triglycerides, and that's because I don't eat sugar or foods that turn into sugar. My thyroid consistently reads in the optimal range, and I found a good supplier for my natural thyroid medicine and ordered a three year supply. Now that I've taken the thyroid issue into my own hands I'm doing better than ever and losing weight easier than ever before. And yes, you can bet your bottom dollar that my thyroid function has improved not only because of my new natural thyroid medicine, but because *I don't eat sugar or foods that turn into sugar*! Wink wink. Kicking the poison called sugar out of your diet is the best thing you can possibly do for yourself. Period. No matter who you are and what health concerns you have, you certainly won't get better if you eat sugar and your body certainly does not need sugar! Limiting carbs is a good idea no matter who you are.

There's an old, outdated myth that claims that the body "requires" carbohydrates for "proper fuel" and especially, they say, for brain function, but that information is very clearly wrong based upon updated information. Yes, the brain requires a certain amount of glucose, but recent studies clearly show that the body prefers dietary fats over glucose for fuel (and low carb diets provide plenty of healthy dietary fats) and it's also a proven fact that the liver has a really easy time converting fats and proteins to glucose. So where is the need for carbs in the diet then? Answer; *there is none.*

Other studies mentioned in this book talk about brain function and the fact that the brain thrives on cholesterol, in other words, healthy animal fats. The brain uses nearly 25% of the body's total cholesterol and people who use *Lipitor* and other cholesterol lowering drugs frequently report memory loss, forgetfulnes, etc. in addition to about 900 or so other "side effects"! Keeping healthy fats reasonably high is definitely your best bet when it comes to the proven science.

Concerning the brain's need for glucose, people who perpetuate the mainstream myth claim that the body requires 130 grams of carbs per day in order to properly feed the brain the necessary amount of glucose, which is blatant nonsense. Pure rubbish. *Not true at all.* First of all, it's definitely not a healthy idea eating all of those carbs every day! Even if you're healthy as a horse that simply isn't wise advice if you desire to remain healthy!

> "During the Paleolithic period, many thousands of years ago, our ancestors ate primarily vegetables, fruit, nuts, roots and meat—and a wide variety of it. This diet was high in fats and protein, and low in grain- and sugar-derived carbohydrates. The average person's diet today, on the other hand, is the complete opposite, and the average person's health is a testament of what happens when you adhere to a faulty diet. Humans today suffer more chronic and debilitating diseases than ever before."

> - Dr. Joseph Mercola

Yes, there are "good fats" and "bad fats". As a general guideline, any fat and/or oil that is 100% natural is a safe and healthy fat to consume. If it has been tampered with by human "technology" and processed in any way shape or form, then it is likely very deadly. And if it has been sitting on the shelf too long it can become rancid, which is also a deadly form of fat. Trans fats such as deep fryer oils are a big killer, beware of french fries and fast "food" you'll die! But eating a big slab of prime rib, a fatty sausage or a big pile of scrambled eggs won't kill you. Those are natural, healthy fats and are not to be feared, but to be embraced! It is only those man made, unnatural fats and old rancid oils that will kill you, not the natural contents of your food! Your body thrives on those fats. Eat them to your heart's content! I do, and my total cholesterol level is normal thank you very much. Sugar and carbs is what raises your cholesterol, not animal fats! *Please do* read the chapter that I've written on cholesterol for more detailed information.

The myth perpetuaters apparently don't know that the liver converts fats to glucose for the purpose of fueling the brain, making it absolutely uneccessary to eat carbs of any kind? The body loves fats more than sugars, and that's a fact folks. As a matter of fact, the body doesn't like sugar. If you look at the results of numerous studies they indicate that sugar is quite literally a poison to the body. Sugar kills and any argument that says that consuming sugar and/or carbs is necessary for proper "health" is a faulty argument that contradicts the scientific facts. Sugar is 100% uneccessary to consume in any form. You'll do just fine without it, I know because I don't eat it and I'm feeling better than ever! My results aren't "anecdotal evidence" because people in general who stop eating sugar experience the same results. They're replicated in patient after patient at the Atkins center as reported in Dr. Atkins' books and they're replicated with pretty much anybody who stops eating sugar and carbs. Keeping carbs low and embracing healthy animal fats is common sense based upon real science.

> "The truth is [that] fat is the preferred fuel of human metabolism and has been for most of human evolution. Under normal human circumstances, we actually require only minimal amounts of glucose, most or all of which can be supplied by the liver as needed on a daily basis. The simple SAD fact that carbs/glucose are so readily available and cheap today doesn't mean that we should depend on them as a primary source of fuel or revere them so highly. In fact, it is this blind allegiance to the 'Carb Paradigm' that has driven so many of us to experience the vast array of metabolic problems that threaten to overwhelm our health care system."
>
> - Mark Sisson, fitness author and blogger, distance runner, triathlete and Ironman competitor. Finished 4th in the February 1982 Ironman World Championship.

The gout condition that I've had to deal with in the past has seemed to vanish, and the deadly MRSA infection that I once had to deal with is gone forever, I've seen no sign of it whatsoever in over two years. I report on all of these battles with my health in this book, and I'm very proud to report that after taking my healthcare and diet plan into my own hands I have succeeded in restoring my health back to normal function, for the most part anyway, and I've done it without the use of drugs and without the help of a so-called "doctor". Drugs cannot and do not promote health, *ever.* They may alleviate certain symptoms, but *at the expense of causing other problems* later in life due to their *toxicity.* The key to health is to *detoxify,* and fortify your nutrients, not to add in more toxins with chemical drugs! Establishment "doctors" are killers, giving people toxic drugs that are totally and completely unnecessary, drugs that cause huge side effects and problems, *when all that is required is proper nutrition (!),* and I am living proof of that, thank you very much. I've succeeded in refraining from allowing myself to be poisoned by establishment "doctors" and I'm no longer complying with their medical system, and the results of that are outstanding. I'll soon be at a weight I've not seen since high school, and all of my previous health conditions including diabetes, hypertension and a deadly MRSA infection have completely stabilized and/or vanished into thin air, no thanks to the establishment's "doctors" and a huge round of applause *to myself* for taking the time to do the research and educate myself. Without that I could easily be dead right now, MRSA is certainly nothing to play with and the establishment's "doctors" offered me absolutely no solution, I had to find it myself! Details in this book.

And that's about it for now. I just wanted to do a casual report on my progress. I am very excited about my results and I hope that more and more people will start to take control of their own lives and their own health through self-education, and I offer this book as a starting place for their journey. I strive to educate because if my work saves even only one life, or makes even only one person's life better, then it was worth it.

Namaste,
Kenneth C. Dyer, Jr.
July 22nd, 2016

Introduction

Beam me up, Scotty, there's no intelligent life on this planet. The common people actually *believe* that they can go to the pharmacy, pick up a prescription drug full of toxic chemicals, put those toxic chemicals into their bodies, and then magically become "healthier" because of it. "It's good for you!" said the doctor. "Here, have some more drugs! These are *good* drugs! And I'm a doctor. Doctors know best. You can trust me!" And the sad thing is that most people are more than willing to comply. "Sure doc, no problem! You're the one with the diploma hanging on the wall! I'll take this drug because you said so! No questions asked! Thank you doctor! Thank you so much! Have a nice day!"

Something is very, very wrong with a society where the majority of people believe such nonsense and follow such lousy advice. We have "doctors" who were sent to school for seven years, sometimes longer, who can't even comprehend the possibility that they are causing the destruction of their patient's health by prescribing toxic drug "treatments" that are **totally unnecessary**. Interestingly, the word pharmaceutical is derived from the Greek words pharmakeia, pharmakeus, pharmakos, pharmakon, etc. which means "sorcery" or *"poisoner"*.

Many, probably most "doctors" of today also lack knowledge concerning the simple basics of nutrition, and what they know about nutritional supplements and herbs is minimal because they're taught very little of that during their indoctrination, I mean "education". With a few exceptions, what they do happen to know in those areas is mainly the biased "science" that they're given by the *American Medical Association*, or the *American Heart Association*, or the *American Diabetes Association*, etc. and most of that information (especially concerning nutrition and diet for diabetic patients) is *misinformation* that actually hurts more than helps patients. We'll be delving into that in great detail in this book.

Prescription drugs kill one person every nineteen minutes in America alone, and that's when they are taken *as directed*. When they're not taken as directed it is largely because "doctors" have gotten the patient addicted to the drugs in the first place, not all of the time, but a good percentage of the time, and as far as I'm concerned "doctors" must be held responsible for that as well.

> "Death by medicine is a twenty-first century epidemic, and America's war on drugs is clearly directed at the wrong enemy."
>
> - Dr. Joseph Mercola

An article appeared in the *Journal of the American Medical Association* on July 26th 2000 entitled *"America's Health Care System is the Third Leading Cause of Death"* by Barbara Starfield, M.D. which states the following:

> "...the medical system has played a large role in undermining the health of Americans. According to several research studies in the last decade, a total of 225,000 Americans per year have died as a result of their medical treatments:
>
> • 12,000 deaths per year due to unnecessary surgery
> • 7000 deaths per year due to medication errors in hospitals
> • 20,000 deaths per year due to other errors in hospitals
> • 80,000 deaths per year due to infections in hospitals
> • 106,000 deaths per year due to negative effects of drugs
>
> Thus, America's healthcare-system-induced deaths are the third leading cause of the death in the U.S., after heart disease and cancer."

Mike Adams, from *NaturalNews.com* sums it up nicely:

> "Western medicine has failed our people. Today, even while prescription drugs are more frequently consumed than ever before in the history of civilization, our nation has skyrocketing rates of obesity and chronic disease. Western medicine simply does not work. It is an outmoded system of medicine dominated by the financial interests of pharmaceutical companies, power-hungry officials at the FDA, and old-school doctors whose myopic view of health prevents them from exploring the true causes of healing. Modern medical schools don't even teach healing or nutrition. No practitioner of western medicine has ever taught me a single thing about being healthy."

Concerning nutritional advice as given by the *US Department of Agriculture* (USDA), which most "doctors" stand by with an iron fist, the public is being hoodwinked. If we travel back in time, say to the 1950s and 1960s and compare those people to the people of today we'll see a glaringly obvious problem. Think of the *Leave It To Beaver* era for a minute. How many obese people did you see? While watching the *Andy Griffith Show* many 300+ lb people did you see? And by way of comparison, when you take a trip to WalMart today how many 350+ pounders do you see rolling around on those electric shopping carts? They're everywhere. Obesity is a national epidemic. A very high percentage of people are obese and diabetes has risen in astonishing numbers. In 1910 heart attacks were virtually nonexistent and only 1 in 100,000 had diabetes. Look at where we're at today! There is a *reason* for that! If you look at the USDA's (in)famous food pyramid, the bottom of it is loaded up with *massive carbohydrates*!

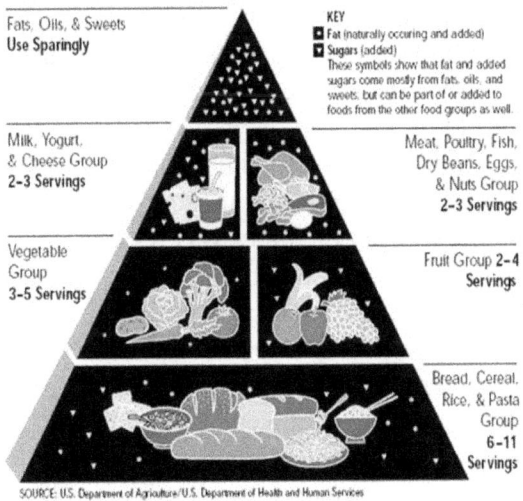

Fats, Oils, & Sweets
Use Sparingly

KEY
■ Fat (naturally occuring and added)
▼ Sugars (added)
These symbols show that fat and added sugars come mostly from fats, oils, and sweets, but can be part of or added to foods from the other food groups as well.

Milk, Yogurt, & Cheese Group
2-3 Servings

Meat, Poultry, Fish, Dry Beans, Eggs, & Nuts Group
2-3 Servings

Vegetable Group
3-5 Servings

Fruit Group 2-4 Servings

Bread, Cereal, Rice, & Pasta Group
6-11 Servings

SOURCE: U.S. Department of Agriculture/U.S. Department of Health and Human Services

And I quote; "Bread, Cereal, Rice & Pasta Group; **6 to 11 servings a day**" is their official recommendation. For those who don't know the basics of nutrition, carbs turn into pure sugar (glucose) in the body after consumption. Carbohydrates raise triglycerides and cholesterol like crazy, blood sugar levels and insulin levels as well as blood pressure levels, and of course they cause weight gain because carbs are pure sugar, yet we're encouraged by the USDA to consume them in mass quantities because those "healthy whole grains" are good for us! Look again at their food pyramid! Insanity! But that's what they recommend. And then they conveniently forget to tell people that two slices of wheat bread will raise blood sugar more than a *Snickers* bar. If you don't believe me, go to *Google.com*, type in "glycemic index" and see for yourself. Wheat bread is rated 72, while *table sugar* is only 59! By comparison, a *Snickers* bar is only 41. In other words the "healthy whole grains" that are recommended by the government are making people fat and giving people diabetes. You're better off with a *Snickers* bar! Yet this is what we're told by the government to eat. And keep in mind that this is *in addition* to the fact that the average American eats *160 pounds of processed sugar* every year! Americans are quite literally killing themselves and the government's recommendations certainly aren't helping one bit. The government is recommending high carb diets to all of the people and claiming that it's "healthy", meanwhile the drug companies are raking in record profits for cholesterol lowering drugs, diabetes drugs, blood pressure drugs, etc. Is that a coincidence? You tell me!

Concerning the FDA's so-called "approval" of various drugs, they keep getting looser and looser. The FDA is answering to the drug companies, not the other way around. It's all about money not safety. Lawsuits, settlements and drug recalls are at an all time high. Commercials on television for drug injury settlements are common these days as well. The FDA claims to "protect" the public and keep the drugs that they approve safe, yet on their very own website, on a page named *"Why Learn about Adverse Drug Reactions (ADR)?"* they *admit to* the following about the drugs that they approve:

"Over 2 MILLION serious ADRs yearly
100,000 DEATHS yearly
ADRs 4th leading cause of death ahead of pulmonary disease, diabetes, AIDS, pneumonia, accidents and automobile deaths
Ambulatory patients ADR rate—unknown
Nursing home patients ADR rate— 350,000 yearly"

The page address is here: *http://www.fda.gov/Drugs/DevelopmentApprovalProcess/ DevelopmentResources/DrugInteractionsLabeling/ucm114848.htm*

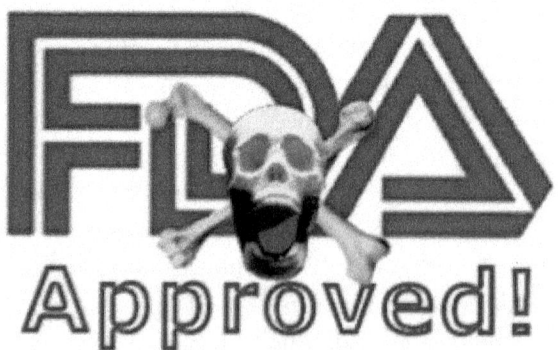

"If al-Qaeda were caught dispensing toxic chemicals disguised as medicine to innocent civilians they would be sent off to Guantanamo Bay without trial and locked away indefinitely. But when the FDA does the very same thing on a much more massive scale nobody bats an eye. And yet the number of people that the FDA has killed with its drugs is far more than the number killed during 911 or the Oklahoma City bombing. The organized crime ring that is the federal government today is the real terrorist threat that we all face on a daily basis. And until the American people collectively wake up to this reality, we will continue to watch her friends, our families and our children, which are the casualties of this ongoing terrorist attack, lay waste at the hands of Big Pharma and the FDA."

- Ethan Huff of *NaturalNews.com*

The medical establishment clearly is not doing its job. That is a simple fact. And that is why I use "quotes" when referring to so-called "doctors" because I do not consider them to be doctors. *Real doctors* promote health. For the most part, the rest of them are just **drug pushers**, earning sales points from drug companies and enjoying luxury cruises to the Bahamas for their drug promotion efforts. The drug companies give them more than adequate incentive to prescribe more drugs. The more they prescribe the more perks they receive, the more income they reap. As a matter of fact, Big Pharma spends $$ *billions* $$ bribing and influencing "doctors":

"The 'Sunshine Act,' a provision of the 2010 Affordable Care Act, intended to create transparency so the public would have access to the nitty-gritty facts about physician payoffs...is now in place and the first report just hit the presses.

One striking fact to emerge from the report is that the amount of money drug companies and medical device manufacturers have been paying to health care providers to snag their allegiance is almost unthinkable. In the five-month period from August through December of last year alone, pharmaceutical companies paid at least $3.5 billion to physicians and teaching hospitals in the United States. That's more than the annual gross national product of Fiji and Bhutan combined. And remember, we're talking about less than half a year's worth of payouts. If the bribery remained at the same level for the entire year, the amount expended would exceed the entire GDP of countries like Afghanistan, Nepal, or Paraguay."

Full article is here: *http://jonbarron.org/doctors-and-drugs/pharmaceutical-payouts#.VSGPA_nF-So*

And I hate to sound like a pessimist, but I really do believe in my heart that a very high percentage of "doctors" are *not* in it for humanity's sake, they're only in it for the big money. They want a life long career and most of them are not willing to sacrifice their careers by rocking the boat and going against the grain. They just quietly go along with the system, ignoring the fact that they're hurting people in the process.

The problem is that the system is rigged. The table is tilted. Banking families (the Rockefellers and the Rothschilds in particular) own and control everything from the food that we eat, to the "educational" institutions that train our "doctors", to the slanted "science" that we're presented with, to the corrupt politicians that are in bed with the drug companies, to the mass media that the drug companies advertise with, and everything in between. Big Pharma not only spends billions on bribing "doctors" they spend billions on advertising. They spend more on advertising than they do on research! Recently there was a survey done of network TV broadcasts and it was determined that some *25% of all commercials* were for prescription drugs such as *Viagra, Claritin, Celebrex, Allegra, Levitra, Zoloft, Cialas, Nexium* and so forth, and so on.

> "The media has many different techniques that they routinely use to brainwash the general public. They can all be summarized in two words: 'whited sepulcher'. They lie, withhold information, deceive you, tell half-truths, and so on...The media are nothing but worthless whores. They sell out to the highest bidder, which is always the corrupt pharmaceutical industry. Everything they say is aimed to please those that pay the most."
>
> - Webster Kehr of *CancerTutor.com*

They also spend billions on lobbying efforts, with over 1300 Big Pharma lobbyists on Capitol Hill, more than two for every member of congress, pushing their agenda onto the American public through a *very cooperative* Federal Government.

We're spoon fed nonsense 24/7 and it's all geared towards one thing. Profits, profits and more profits. Profits for drug companies, mainly. Drugs are big money. Drugs are a multi-billion dollar a year industry. Illegal drugs are chump change compared to Big Pharma. With an empire like that do you think they want cures? The last thing they want is to lose sales. Every cure represents lost customers and lost sales.

Something is very, very wrong with this so-called system of "health" when you turn on your TV and see commercials for drugs, and when they get to the end of the commercial they drone on for 5 minutes about all of the possible side effects! "May cause bleeding from the asshole, may cause a third arm to grow out of your forehead, may cause green pus to come out of your eye socket...." and on and on! This is health care? Here's one; *may cause people with intelligence to tell the drug companies where to go*!

As for the science behind their miracle drugs, mainstream "medicine" isn't based upon science *at all* because only about 12% of its drugs and treatments are proven effective. Yes, you read that correctly. *Only about 12% of most commonly prescribed drugs are proven effective.* Researchers working with the *British Medical Journal* looked at 2500 of the most commonly prescribed drugs, measuring effectiveness vs. harmful side effects. To determine that a drug is effective, the researchers had to find *just one* study involving a single group of people that demonstrated a *benefit greater than any harm* recorded by the participants. The researchers found that, at the very most, only 12% of the 2500 drugs studied have met that one simple criteria. In other words 88% of all the drugs studied *do more harm than good.* For more info on this all you need to do is order a copy of the *British Medical Association's* annual *Clinical Evidence Handbook: The International Source Of The Best Available Evidence For Effective Health Care* and see the data for yourself.

One of Big Pharma's main methods of promoting drugs to doctors is, of course, those "prestigious" medical journals that all "doctors" love to read for furthering indoctrination, I mean "education". Most people trust those journals, "doctors" certainly do, but the fact of the matter is that **blatant fraud** is a very common occurrence in those journals.

In 1987, the *New England Journal of Medicine* ran an article following the research of Dr. R. Slutsky. Over a 7 year period he published 137 articles in several "peer-reviewed" medical journals and it was proven that **60** of those articles featured blatant *lies* and *fraud.*

In 2010 Dr. Scott Reuben plead guilty to publishing dozens of *fake* research studies in medical journals. A *fake* study of one drug, in particular, Celebrex, was the topic of many of those articles. Hundreds of "doctors" quoted his *fake* research as evidence for the efficacy of the drug in numerous medical journals. As it turns out there were no patients enrolled in that study! He *faked* the whole thing! The same guy also *faked* studies on Vioxx, a drug that even the FDA admits caused over 50,000 deaths. Reuben had been *faking* data for over 13 years and published 10 fake "scientific" papers and 21 articles in "peer-reviewed" medical journals.

And that's what happens when the original "study" is a fraud, it creates a domino effect where the original lie gets quoted hundreds of times, and innocent people end up getting hurt and killed all in the name of *profits for drug companies*. And I really hate to break the news to you (wait, no I don't!), but drug companies engage in fake "studies" all the time. Dr. Slutsky and Dr. Reuben are merely two examples of hundreds. I only mentioned them to make my point, and that is that *fraud in medical journals is rampant*.

> "It is simply no longer possible to believe much of the clinical research that is published, or to rely on the judgment of trusted physicians or authoritative medical guidelines. I take no pleasure in this conclusion, which I reached slowly and reluctantly over my two decades as an editor of the *New England Journal of Medicine*."
>
> - Marcia Angell

The Institute for Evidence Based Medicine did a study recently that found that 94% of the promotional literature sent to "doctors" has no scientific basis whatsoever.

> "Pharmaceutical companies engage in mass scientific fraud in order to distort their studies and get drugs approved based upon rather shaky science, but what surprises me about this new research is the extent of it: 94% of the marketing claims are unsubstantiated and unsupported by scientific evidence. That's an alarming number – it means **19 of 20** statements made by drug companies in their marketing literature are false."
>
> - Mike Adams of *NaturalNews.com*

In other words, they lie their asses off in the name of profits and they don't care who they hurt in the process. *Money comes first, innocent and unsuspecting, every day normal people come last.*

Dr. Richard Horton, editor-in-chief of *The Lancet*, one of the most respected peer-reviewed medical journals in the world recently published an interesting statement:

> "The case against science is straightforward: much of the scientific literature, perhaps half, may simply be untrue. Afflicted by studies with small sample sizes, tiny effects, invalid exploratory analysis, and flagrant conflicts of interest, together with an obsession for pursuing fashionable trends of dubious importance, science has taken a turn towards darkness."

In July of 2012, two former employees of *Merck* (the drug company) filed a federal lawsuit against their ex-employer stating that *Merck* had falsified test data trying to make it look like their vaccines were more effective by spiking the blood test with animal antibodies.

Also in July of 2012 *GlaxoSmithKline* plead guilty to bribery, fraud, falsifying drug safety data and lying to the FDA, and agreed to pay one billion in criminal fines and two billion in civil fines following a nine-year federal investigation. According to official sources they routinely bribed "doctors" with high priced vacations and speaking dates.

> "It would be nice to think of medical journals as these bastions of truth and light that have no bias, but in fact, they're businesses, and they make their money, in many cases, from drug company advertisement, and also from sales of the glossy reprints of drug favorable articles to industry. And interestingly, several former editors and chiefs of major medical journals, Richard Horton of 'The *Lancet*', and also a couple of former editors-in-chief of the '*New England Journal of Medicine*' have written books and opined heavily on the favorable impact of drug company influence on medical publishing. There are strong conflicts by the journal to publish drug company favorable articles in order to reap those hundred thousand dollars or so in reprint sales for the favorable articles, and also to keep the drug companies happy so that they continue to get drug company advertising."

- Dr. Beatrice Golomb

Speaking of "drug company advertising", Big Pharma pays for 90% of all of the advertising space in those journals! Dr. Richard Horton of the *The Lancet* puts it bluntly:

> "Journals have devolved into information-laundering operations for the pharmaceutical industry."

I'll be discussing a lot of suppressed information in this book. Information that *they* don't want you to know because it would hurt their precious profit margins. Suppressed yet scientifically proven cures for cancer will be discussed and you will be shocked at how many proven methods there are. Allow me to repeat myself: I said *proven* cures. These cures are suppressed by the mainstream because they don't want to lose their precious profits. Cancer is big business! A cure? What's that? We didn't see any cure! Nope, not us!

There is a doctor by the name of Stanislaw Burzynski who was taken to court by the FDA and threatened with up to 290 years in prison and 18.5 million in fines for doing what? For *curing* cancer. Yes, that's right. He was *curing cancer,* and the FDA accused him of using methods that were not properly "approved" by them, and of course, they won't approve it because they deny that there is any evidence that it really cures cancer, never mind that he has a 60% overall success rate over a period of 40 years! It's as corrupt as corrupt can get. Details are in this book. And so are many other interesting little tidbits of information concerning your immoral, criminal, *for profit* "health care" system.

Don't misunderstand me here. I'm not trying to demonize

all doctors, or slam the medical industry as a whole. They aren't all bad. Dr. Robert Atkins was a great man and so is Dr. Joseph Mercola. Dr. William Davis and Dr. Michael Murray are pretty cool too. There are many doctors who embrace natural treatments first and foremost (as it should be) and who don't allow themselves to be sellouts for Big Pharma bribes, perks and payouts, but those doctors are rare, and they take a lot of flack, ridicule and abuse from the mainstream because they *rightly* go against the grain. Those doctors know that drugs should only be used in cases of emergencies when no other options exist, and as far as I'm concerned if doctors aren't doing that then they aren't doctors, they are drug pushers, nothing more. Which is, again, why I use quotes when referring to "doctors". They're not.

But despite the corruption and criminal behavior of the *American Murder Association*, I mean *American Medical Association*, if I was bleeding to death or having a heart attack the first place you'd see me run to is the emergency room! I certainly wouldn't run to an herbalist! No way. My ass would be at the hospital allowing mainstream medicine to save my life. And that's what I believe the function of the medical establishment should be. *Emergency care*. When it comes to diet and nutrition and everyday health concerns, when it comes to health *maintenance*, I very firmly believe in the novel idea and concept of *personal responsibility*. Yes, that's right! I believe that all people should take an active role in their own health care and accept *personal responsibility* for it. Pretty radical huh? But it makes all the sense in the world, because eating Twinkies and drinking Coca-Cola all day long and then running to the "doctor" for a magic pill that will "fix" you when you get type 2 diabetes just isn't an option. Do you see it working? I certainly don't. I see fat people everywhere, and people dying from prescription drugs left and right. We must accept *personal responsibility*!

The first section of this book will consist of my personal story in regards to my experiences with "doctors" and what I've learned through my own research about how to take care of myself without their worthless "care". I've been through some terrible health problems in my life including weight problems, type 2 diabetes, gout, damaged knees, psoriasis, MRSA infection, high blood pressure, hypothyroidism and high triglycerides/cholesterol and "doctors" have been of no help to me whatsoever. For the most part they've been worthless and because of that I was forced to do *my own research*. I am proud to say that I have mastered all of my health problems *without* their "help" and *without* using a single drug.

I have modified my diet and adopted a protocol of herbs and natural supplements to *control all aspects of my health* and I am living proof that drugs aren't necessary to be healthy, even in the midst of very serious health concerns like mine! Truth be told, in most cases drugs only do more damage. The genius suggestion that you'll be healthier if you fill your body with toxic drugs is exactly the same as saying that filling a helium balloon with lead will make it float better! There is simply no place for toxins in a healthy body. Period.

You're probably wondering if I'm opposed to all drugs. No, I'm not. I do believe that in cases of emergencies drugs are sometimes necessary. I'm a firm believer in natural methods, but I'm not insanely fanatical about it. If I was all banged up in a car crash, I'd happily welcome some pain killers and whatever else is necessary to get me back on my feet again. Drugs are fine for *temporary emergency type situations if it's totally necessary*, but when it comes to everyday *maintenance* drugs are simply no option and I certainly don't believe in them, not even for a second. *Why would any intelligent person prefer drugs when there are safe, natural and side effect free treatments available?* You'd have to be as dumb as a stump to choose toxic drugs when it's not necessary. There is an interesting thing that I do, it's called *thinking*, and common sense says to *use the least harmful treatment available*. Using a drug when you can use a safe and natural supplement instead is an exercise in either ignorance or stupidity, or both. Unfortunately, the common people don't realize that so many natural alternatives to drugs are out there and "doctors" certainly won't tell them. "Doctors" only do one thing, for the most part; **push drugs** and *that* is precisely why I am writing this book, to *educate* innocent people who don't know about natural alternatives, so that they can be aware what their **real options** are, instead of just taking lousy advice from their "doctor".

As I mentioned earlier, the majority of the advice that I have received from "doctors" has proven worthless. In a way I am thankful for that because it forced me to research and find my own solutions and act as my own personal naturopathic physician. I am now feeling very empowered with the knowledge that I have accumulated, and now I don't feel that I have to rely on other people as much. It got real tiresome and annoying, having a problem, going to the "doctor" and being given an ineffective solution, or simply being given a prescription for toxic drugs and being told to have a nice day. It got to the point where I was thinking "Don't you ever do anything besides push drugs?"

Had I allowed my health care to be under the directive of the mainstream medical establishment, I would most definitely be extremely obese, shooting insulin three times a day and on four or more prescription drugs. I would be *far from healthy* if I had chosen to listen to them, and the sad thing is that millions of people *are* listening to them! Do yourselves a favor; *read this book!*

This book will cover the details of the *American Diabetes Association's* recommended diet for all diabetic patients, which destroys the health of millions. I will also discuss my own personal diet, which not only basically cured my type 2 diabetes (as long as I continue the diet) but also works for all *other aspects of general health*, and there are scientific studies to prove it.

As for my MRSA infection, there's no telling what would have happened had I not found an effective cure through my own personal research. I battled that problem for a good year before I finally nipped it in the bud with an amazing supplement that you can buy at any health food store. (Details inside this book).

I'll be discussing nutritional supplements, herbs and alternatives to prescription drugs extensively. The German government utilizes herbs into their mainstream medicine, prescribing herbs the same way "doctors" in America prescribe drugs. Their equivalent of our FDA is called the *German E Commission* and they have a reference book similar to the PDR (*Physician's Desk Reference*) and it's called *The German E Commission Monographs*. If you are skeptical and require scientific evidence for herbal treatments, please refer to this manual. Other great sources of science behind supplements and herbs are *HerbMed.org* and *GreenMedInfo.com*. Additionally, *Scholar.Google.com* and *PubMed.gov* are websites that have millions of entries with the scientific studies for virtually any supplement you can think of, herbs included. Simply go to the websites and type in your inquiry.

I'll supply you with a list of suggested reading and films to watch at the end of the book, and suggested websites will be contained throughout the book. In other words, herbs and nutritional healing methods aren't "quackery" they are backed by real science, *unlike the vast majority of all chemical drugs* as I've shown above. The mainstream establishment has succeeded in keeping their little secrets for a long time, but in the day and age of the internet I'm afraid their party is soon over. They won't be able to keep a lid on the numerous cures for cancer for very much longer, and they'll be forced to admit that and many other things.

I'll also be discussing facts about vaccines and the sudden rise in autism and sudden infant death syndrome as they keep giving children more and more vaccines. I'll discuss HIV/AIDS facts, ADHD facts and drugs like Ritalin, proven cancer cures and other topics related to health care.

My goal in writing this book is simply to help as many people as I possibly can, and *wake people up* to the reality of the drugged up, brainwashed and *profit making* culture that we all live in. I want you to know that you don't have to take drugs to be healthy, as a matter of fact, *you can't be healthy if you take drugs*, that's impossible! The key to health is *nutrition* and nutritional supplements and herbs play a major role in that.

I hope that all of you take this information and use it to your advantage. I hope that you all adopt natural healing techniques for yourselves and start "just saying no to drugs", and I hope that you pass this information along to everyone that you know. Last but not least, I hope that you and your loved ones enjoy a life full of positive energy, joy, peace, love and above all fantastic health in mind, body and spirit.

Namaste,
Kenneth C. Dyer, Jr.

Part One:
My Personal Health History

In the beginning there was health. I was young, full of energy, and I had no idea what hypothyroidism was. I had no knowledge of type 2 diabetes, I had never heard of high blood pressure or cholesterol. And gout? What's that? Superbugs like MRSA didn't even exist back then, so I knew nothing of them either, but I would know about all of these things from personal experience later in life, plus much more.

I never had any reason to mistrust "doctors", I pretty much assumed that they knew what they were doing. My Mom would take me to the "doctor" and they seemed nice enough. I always thought that they had my best interests in mind. I was young, I was healthy and I was ignorant. Only later in life did I figure out that my best interests are irrelevant and that only the interests of the drug companies are considered. Sure, there are many doctors out there with good intentions, but sadly they are misinformed and indoctrinated into the system and if they buck the system or go against the grain they lose their licenses, get threatened with jail by the FDA, etc.

I had not received a decent education from my parents on health matters. My Dad didn't care about his health, never went to the "doctor" and as a result he and I never discussed those things, at least not until much later in life when I was an adult. Shortly before he passed away, Dad took an interest in his health, but unfortunately it was too late. Mom was a "doctor person", but her lifestyle was far from healthy. Her influence on me was definitely not healthy either. She was always buying sweets and offering "Big Gulps" and McDonalds on a regular basis. I never thought about it when I was younger but now I can see that I am diabetic because I was never properly educated on nutrition and my parents were a lousy example to follow. I was taught an extremely unhealthy lifestyle by my parents.

Inevitably, as I grew older the health problems slowly started creeping in. Due to my ignorance and feelings of invincibility, and my extremely unhealthy diet, my lifestyle started catching up with me. I was no longer healthy.

Hypothyroidism

My first big problem was my metabolic state, followed by loss of energy and weight gain. I was only in my early 20s and already I was diagnosed with hypothyroidism, which is basically a slow metabolism due to a sluggish thyroid gland. The "doctors" had put me on *Levothyroxine*, a synthetic hormone replacement drug, and I did ok on that for quite some time, until I hit my early 40s, and then it started to fail me. They gave me bigger and bigger doses but I was still tired, still irritable, and still unable to make it through the day without a mid-afternoon nap.

About six months ago, in September of 2014, I wanted to find an independent solution to my thyroid issues rather than having to constantly go into "doctor" offices for prescription refills once every three months. I had felt for a long time that "doctors" are incompetent and I knew that the care that I was receiving was inadequate, but I still went because I desperately needed my thyroid medicine. My last visit to the "doctor" was totally unacceptable and I was very angry. The "doctor" had left me on a dose of thyroid that was too weak according to my lab results. According to their *very own standards*, my results were *very clearly* out of range and a higher dose was required, but she left it the same! My anger served as a great catalyst because it gave me much incentive to find my own solution. I was determined to break loose once and for all, and so I began scouring the internet like mad. I had been searching for thyroid solutions for three days straight when I stumbled upon a fantastic website that turned everything around for me. I had finally found my solution!

For those of you with hypothyroidism, here is your life saving website; *StopTheThyroidMadness.com*. The owner and operator of the website, Janie Bowthorpe, is one awesome lady! I have learned so much from her, and I am extremely grateful for her efforts. A thyroid patient herself, also frustrated with "doctors" and their inadequate care, she began to branch off on her own. During her research she decided to open this website, and compile all of the information to this patient ran website, a community of thyroid patients helping thyroid patients, sharing knowledge, experiences and information. Through the power of the internet, Janie managed to create a very scholarly website. The information and knowledge that I have received from her website and the book of the same title, which is based on the information from the website, has enabled me to know more about thyroid problems than just about any "doctor". My Mom is a thyroid patient as well, and she sees a "thyroid specialist". When she tells me what he is saying to her it is clear that he doesn't know much. It's also *very clear* to me that I know more than he does thanks to Janie's book and website. And that's quite typical among "doctors". They don't know much. They're robots. They're "repeaters" simply repeating and regurgitating what the establishment has "taught" them. These "doctors" are a dime a dozen, and no, their diplomas don't impress me. Seven years of indoctrination while being fed misinformation is nothing for me to be impressed about. Real *doctors* are very rare, but they do exist, and it is *they* who I have tremendous respect for.

The first thing that I learned from Janie is that the TSH (*Thyroid Stimulating Hormone*) lab test that **medication dosages are based upon** is an **inaccurate measure** of thyroid function. It's not quite as simple as checking the TSH level and then adjusting the medication dose based upon that reading! First of all, the TSH hormone isn't even a thyroid hormone, it's a pituitary hormone. The only thing that TSH has to do with thyroid is that it's a *signal to the thyroid* (from the pituitary gland) to release more thyroxine. If the thyroid isn't getting the message or releasing enough thyroxine the pituitary gland will keep sending out the signal, and then you'll see a lab test with a high amount of TSH. If the TSH level is above a certain marker, then hypothyroidism is diagnosed. Granted, a build up of TSH in the system is indeed an effective way to diagnose a sluggish thyroid, but when it comes to dosage levels of medication it's not efficient at all. Many people show lab results that are "in range" yet they still experience terrible symptoms of hypothyroidism. These symptoms include (as copied directly from Janie's website):

- Less stamina than others
- Less energy than others
- Long recovery period after any activity
- Inability to hold children for very long
- Arms feeling like dead weights after activity
- Chronic Low Grade Depression
- Suicidal Thoughts
- Often feeling cold
- Cold hands and feet

- High or rising cholesterol
- Heart disease
- Palpitations
- Fibrillation
- Plaque buildup
- Bizarre and Debilitating reaction to exercise
- Hard stools
- Constipation
- Candida
- No eyebrows or thinning outer eyebrows
- Dry Hair
- Hair Loss
- White hairs growing in
- No hair growth, breaks faster than it grows
- Dry cracking skin
- Nodding off easily
- Requires naps in the afternoon
- Sleep Apnea (which can also be associated with low cortisol)
- Air Hunger (feeling like you can't get enough air)
- Inability to concentrate or read long periods of time
- Forgetfulness
- Foggy thinking
- Inability to lose weight
- Always gaining weight
- Weight loss (a small minority experience this)
- Inability to function in a relationship with anyone
- NO sex drive
- Failure to ovulate and/or constant bleeding
- Moody periods
- PMS
- Inability to get pregnant; miscarriages
- Excruciating pain during period
- Nausea
- Swelling/edema/puffiness
- Aching bones/muscles
- Osteoporosis
- Bumps on legs
- Acne on face and in hair
- Breakout on chest and arms
- Hives
- Exhaustion in every dimension–physical, mental, spiritual, emotional
- Inability to work full-time
- Inability to stand on feet for long periods
- Complete lack of motivation
- Slowing to a snail's pace when walking up slight grade
- Extremely crabby, irritable, intolerant of others
- Handwriting nearly illegible
- Internal itching of ears
- Broken/peeling fingernails
- Dry skin or snake skin
- Major anxiety/worry
- Ringing in ears
- Lactose Intolerance
- Inability to eat in the mornings
- Joint pain
- Carpal tunnel symptoms
- No Appetite
- Fluid retention to the point of Congestive Heart Failure

- Swollen legs that prevented walking
- Blood Pressure problems
- Varicose Veins
- Dizziness from fluid on the inner ear
- Low body temperature
- Raised temperature
- Tightness in throat; sore throat
- Swollen lymph glands
- Allergies (which can also be a result of low cortisol–common with hypothyroid patients)
- Headaches and Migraines
- Sore feet (plantar fascitis); painful soles of feet
- Tailbone pain
- now how do I put this one politely....a cold bum, butt, derriere, fanny, gluteus maximus, haunches, hindquarters, posterior, rear, and/or cheeks.
- Colitis
- irritable bowel syndrome
- painful bladder
- Extreme hunger, especially at nighttime
- Dysphagia (nerve damage causing inability to swallow fluid, food, saliva; can also be caused by a goiter or anxiety)

Obviously many of these symptoms can be caused by problems other than hypothyroidism, but hypothyroid patients commonly complain of these things. My personal symptoms were fatigue, irritability, depression, dry skin, lower than normal body temperature, brain fog/forgetfulness, and a few others.

So if the TSH blood test isn't an adequate assessment of thyroid function, then what is? Well, it's a fairly complex issue and the vast majority of mainstream "doctors" *don't have a clue* as to what's going on. Again, most of them simply check the TSH and adust the medication dosage according to that.

First of all, all thyroid patients should have their *adrenal* function tested, because *adrenal* issues and thyroid issues go together. If you have a thyroid problem the entire endocrine system needs to be looked at, not just the thyroid! As a thyroid patient I never knew that, because in all the 25+ years of being a thyroid patient I never once had one "doctor" mention the adrenal glands to me, or run tests in that area. All they ever did was check the TSH and raise or lower meds according to that number, which is enough to make my blood pressure rise now that I am more educated on thyroid problems. How stupid, negligent and totally incompetent can they be?

The adrenal glands release the hormone cortisol therefore checking those levels is recommended before you start blaming it all on the thyroid alone. The test that Janie recommends is a four-part saliva test. Saliva is the most accurate method, and doing it in four parts makes it possible to track cortisol levels throughout the entire day, from morning until bedtime. If you ask for a cortisol levels test, don't accept any other kind of test, because the other options aren't sufficient. Repeat: *four-part saliva* test for cortisol levels! If your cortisol levels are out of whack then obviously that issue needs to be addressed in addition to the thyroid.

Something else very important to thyroid function are iron levels. You need to have those checked. In particular, you need to have your ferritin (reserve iron) levels checked. If your iron is low, then obviously that issue needs addressed in addition to the thyroid.

Other than the TSH, cortisol and ferritin levels, you'll also need to check the Free T4 (FT4), Free T3 (FT3) and Reverse T3 (RT3) levels. The FT4 is the amount of available T4 hormone that you have floating around in your blood stream, and the FT3 is the amount of free T3. Reverse T3 is a hormone that works to cancel out the efficiency of T3, which is the active hormone that gives you your energy, therefore knowing that number is also very important. With an optimally functioning thyroid the TSH should be at the bottom of the standard range (0.35 - 5.50 mIU/ml), the FT4 should be at the middle of the standard range (0.9 - 2 ng/dl), and the FT3 should be at the top of the standard range (2.0 - 4.4 ng/dl). There is a formula to calculate your RT3 ratio. See Janie's website or book for complete details.

There are numerous other tests that need to be conducted and sometimes thyroid issues can be very complex, but I wanted to make sure that I gave you a crash course on the basics in this book. A whole book would be required for me to address all that needs to be addressed on this issue, so I'll just leave that to Janie by referring you to her website and book. She spells it all out for you in plain English, easy to understand, and tells you everything that you need to know.

Janie's website helped me to realize that the medication that I was on, *levothyroxine*, was very inferior, which explains why it didn't work for me very well when I started getting into my 40s.

The thyroid gland actually puts out five different hormones (T4, T3, T2, T1 and calcitonin) not just one, and those hormones work together synergistically. The medication that I was on only included the one known as T4. These synthetic "T4 only" medications cause a lot of problems for people because they don't offer the full spectrum, they rob the patient of the synergistic properties of the hormones that the thyroid makes. As for T4, it is a secondary hormone which has to be converted into the active hormone, T3. When "doctors" prescribe T4 only medications, the patient's body has to be able to convert that into T3 and many people have problems with that. T3 is the hormone that gives you your energy. If your body can't convert T4 into T3 then you're basically screwed.

The medication that I am now on, which is recommended by Janie Bowthorpe, is *natural desiccated thyroid* (NDT) and I feel 100% better! I feel like a new person! Most NDT is powdered thyroid gland from pigs (porcine), but there are bovine (cows) varieties too. NDT gives your body *exactly* what your body would be making, the five hormones listed above; T4, T3, T2, T1 and calcitonin. Contrary to what many ignorant doctors will tell you, it is produced with very strict guidelines and standards, and dosages are scientifically calculated per tablet, as a matter of fact there are prescription brands available. The most popular kind is *Armour.* The brand that I use is called *Thyroid-S* and it is available without a prescription. This brand is from Thailand, but it is available for order out of Los Angeles, CA at this website: *NDThyroid.com*. As someone with experience, I can tell you that the *Thyroid-S* brand without a prescription is by far the best way to go because you can control your own dosage as well as bypass the doctor's office every three months for refills. When I ordered *Thyroid-S* it was sent to me with a paper from the lab showing the exact measurements of thyroid hormone that were detected in the batch when it was tested for quality standards. This is a very high quality product from a very professional lab, nothing to worry about at all. I was a bit skeptical at first, but then I read numerous reports on Janie's website from thyroid patients who were very happy with it.

When it comes to lab tests, Janie has a list of websites where you can order your own and then go to the local lab of your choice to get your blood drawn. That's what I do now that I've sworn off all "doctors". That way I can monitor my dosage appropriately, and I am proud to say that my numbers are currently perfect. Much better than they were before when I was under the care of a "doctor" and stuck putting up with appointments once every three months, pharmacy visits, etc.

Other brands of NDT that don't require a prescription include *Thiroyd* (yes, that's how it's spelled) and that's out of Thailand as well, from a different company. I've read good reports on this one too, but from what I've read it does appear as if *Thyroid-S* is just a little bit better. *Thyroid-S* seems to have better binding and holds up longer than *Thiroyd* according to the reports I've read.

Another brand of NDT is *Thyro-Gold* which is available at *NaturalThyroidSolutions.com*. This is an American source.

Lastly, there is *Nutri-Meds*, also an American source and the website is *Nutri-Meds.com*. But again, I do highly recommend *Thyroid-S* because it works like a champ for myself and I've read more positive reviews on this brand than any other. Have I read any negative reviews on these products? Not really, they all seem to be pretty workable products. The only thing that I've heard is that *Nutri-Meds* might not be as potent as the others, but nobody has ever said that it doesn't work. It just seems that maybe they need to take more of it, that's all.

Now that you have the basic rundown and the truth concerning the ineffective methods of the mainstream medical establishment on hypothyroid issues, you might be considering making the switch to NDT (natural desiccated thyroid). Depending upon your condition, this needs to be done with a proper amount of care. The first thing to do, before anything else, is get the "big two" tests; *ferritin* (reserve iron) and *cortisol*. Before you make the switch to NDT you need to make sure that those are at appropriate levels because if you don't check, and if you have low iron or cortisol issues, then you could have unpleasant reactions to the NDT because your body is not yet accustomed to receiving the synergistic blend of thyroid hormones or the direct T3, especially if you've been on a T4 only medication for a long time, and NDT can reveal problems that you have with your adrenal glands and your iron levels. Adrenal or iron issues can get in the way of making a successful switch to NDT, therefore check those *first!* Details are on Janie's website or in her book *Stop the Thyroid Madness*.

After you've verified proper iron/ferritin and cortisol levels, you're safe to go ahead and make the switch to NDT. Do this very slowly. The reason for this is because your body needs time to adjust and get used to receiving the synergistic blend of hormones again, especially if you've been on T4 only meds for many years. The standard recommended procedure is to start at a very low dose, and work up. For example, start at one half "grain" and stay there for a week, and then move up to one grain. Do this week after week, moving up by a half grain until you've reached a point where you no longer feel symptoms of hypothyroidism. When your energy levels feel ok and when your symptoms start clearing up you'll know you've found your optimal dosage.

I personally started out on one grain. I knew that I'd require four or five grains, so I tried one grain at first, for a week and when I didn't experience any unpleasant reactions after one week I moved it up to two grains and my body handled that just fine. When I got up to three grains I noticed some minor queasiness and a tad bit of nausea, but it quickly went away within a couple of days. I did three and one half grains for about a week, felt no unpleasant reactions but still felt like I needed more, so I moved it up to four and stayed there. One month after I started on four grains a day I got my blood tested. My numbers were perfect. So when it comes to adjusting your dosage, use your intuition and pay attention to how you feel, that's the main thing. And then verify it later at the lab.

Now that we've seen that natural thyroid replacement is far, far superior to their synthetic drugs, I'd like to address additional supplements and herbs that are beneficial to thyroid function. I will provide you with a nice list of supplements that benefit thyroid function.

The first thing that you should know is that thyroxine, the hormone that the thyroid glands produce, is literally made of a combination of *iodine* and the amino acid *l-tyrosine*. An excellent and inexpensive source of iodine is *kelp*. L-tyrosine is also fairly inexpensive. Both are available at any health food store. Keep an eye on your blood pressure while taking l-tyrosine if you have a history of high blood pressure. I personally had to discontinue that supplement due the fact that it was raising my blood pressure.

The below supplements work together in many bodily processes, including the manufacture of thyroid hormone. A deficiency in any of these could inhibit thyroid function:

- B-Complex Vitamins
- Selenium
- Vitamin A
- Vitamin E
- Vitamin C
- Zinc

Other beneficial supplements include:

- Ashwaganda
- Bacopa
- Bladderwrack
- Bugleweed
- Copper
- DHEA (very commonly low in people with hypothyroidism)
- Echinacea
- Evening Primrose
- Fish Oils
- Flaxseed
- Ginseng
- Grape Seed Extract
- Lemon Balm
- Licorice Root
- Myrrh
- Pine Bark Extract
- Vitamin D
- Yerba Mate

You're also going to want to make sure that you're taking a high potency multi-vitamin and mineral supplement. I personally also take a trace mineral supplement. The idea of holistic health is to eliminate any and all potential deficiencies, because deficiencies cause disease, therefore you want to cover all your bases. It might require taking numerous supplements, but would you rather take toxic drugs that only lead to further health problems? I personally take three large handfuls of nutritional supplements and herbs daily. Maintaining a healthy diet is mandatory, but the fact remains that you cannot get all of the nutrients that your body requires through diet alone. My supplements keep me in good health and they keep me away from people that I don't want to deal with, namely "doctors". Three handfuls of supplements a day keeps the "doctor" away.

Gout (and Other Forms of Arthritis)

My next big health concern snuck up on me, out of the blue, in the middle of the night, when I was in my late 20s. I was due to be at work that morning, and I felt fine when I went to bed, but when I woke up my foot felt like it was broken. It was swollen to almost twice its normal size and it was so sensitive that I cried out in pain if I even did so much as rub a bed sheet up against it. I was baffled. "What could this be?" I thought. I immediately called my boss to let him know the situation, and then I hopped on one foot out to my car and headed for the emergency room. When I came in the nurse offered me a wheel chair and asked me what the problem was. I said that it felt like my foot was broken, but that I hadn't sustained any injuries, it had crept up on me during the night. She took one look at it and immediately said "that's gout."

Gout is a condition where the blood builds up too much uric acid, and then forms sharp and painful crystals, usually in and around the big toe areas or the feet, and in severe cases in the knees, elbows and other joints, which causes flair-ups similar to rheumatoid arthritis, only far more painful. That morning was the beginning of a struggle with a condition that plagued me on and off for many years.

"Doctors" have standard methods for dealing with gout as they do for everything, and I received the standard treatment. When I left the emergency room I had two prescriptions. One was for a drug called *Colchicine* and the other was called *Allopurinol*. Before I continue I'd like to discuss these drugs.

Colchicine is derived from a quite literally *poisonous* plant named *Colchicum Autumnale*, also known as *Autumn Crocus* or *Meadow Saffron*. The following is a quote from *ThePoisonReview.com*'s website:

> "Colchicine is a feared poison - it impairs the function of cellular microtubules, interfering with essential processes such as mitosis, secretion, protein synthesis, and myocardial function. Even small doses can result in multi-organ failure, and no antidote is available. Onset of life-threatening toxicity can be heralded by \ severe gastrointestinal symptoms."

Full article is here: *http://www.thepoisonreview.com/2010/07/04/colchicine-be-afraid-be-very-afraid/#sthash.aCgkmwg8.dpuf*

Drugs.com states the following on its entry for the *Autumn Crocus* plant:

> "All parts are highly toxic. It may produce severe gastric distress, shock, and inhibit normal cell growth."

> "The entire plant is toxic, primarily because of the colchicine content. After ingestion, immediate burning of the mouth and throat is followed by intense thirst, nausea, and vomiting. Abdominal pain and persistent diarrhea attributed to disturbance of water and electrolyte balance develop because of small and large intestine mucosal lining damage."

> "Veterinary poisonings have been associated with autumn crocus; these often are observed in grazing animals. There have been reports of calves becoming intoxicated by drinking milk from cows that have ingested the plant."

> "There have been reports of children becoming intoxicated by drinking milk from cows that have ingested the plant."

> **Full article is here**: *http://www.drugs.com/npp/autumn-crocus.html*

I mentioned *PubMed.gov* in my introduction concerning them being such a fine source of science behind millions of various supplements. I'd like to share something that I learned there concerning colchicine. The article entitled *"Colchicine: The Dark Side of an Ancient Drug"* states:

> "Colchicine is excreted into breast milk..."

> "Colchicine is used mainly for the treatment and prevention of gout and for familial Mediterranean fever (FMF). It has a narrow therapeutic index, with no clear-cut distinction between nontoxic, toxic, and lethal doses, causing substantial confusion among clinicians. Although colchicine poisoning is sometimes intentional, unintentional toxicity is common and often associated with a poor outcome."

> "Colchicine's toxicity is an extension of its mechanism of action - binding to tubulin and disrupting the microtubular network. As a result, affected cells experience impaired protein assembly, decreased endocytosis and exocytosis, altered cell morphology, decreased cellular motility, arrest of mitosis, and interrupted cardiac myocyte conduction and contractility. The culmination of these mechanisms leads to multi-organ dysfunction and failure."

> "Colchicine poisoning presents in three sequential and usually overlapping phases: 1) 10-24 hrs after ingestion - gastrointestinal phase mimicking gastroenteritis may be absent after intravenous administration; 2) 24 hrs to 7 days after ingestion - multi-organ dysfunction. Death results from rapidly progressive multi-organ failure and sepsis. Delayed presentation, pre-existing renal or liver impairment are associated with poor prognosis. 3) Recovery typically occurs within a few weeks of ingestion, and is generally a complete recovery barring complications of the acute illness."

> **Full article is here**: *http://www.ncbi.nlm.nih.gov/pubmed/20586571*

I don't know about you, but had I known these things at the time there is simply no way that I would have taken that drug. Of course "doctors" never tell you the truth about what they give you, because most likely they don't even know it themselves. All they ever say is that it will "help your condition" because that is what they are indoctrinated and programmed to do. They know that they're supposed to pass out this drug for this problem, that drug for that problem, and so on and so forth. But rarely do they know the real truth about what they're passing out, because as I illustrated in the introduction, their sources of information about drugs are full of lies and fraud. Yes, *Colchicine* does aid in bringing down symptoms of gout, but as you can see, the toxic trade-off is enormous!

And let's not forget how expensive this poison is! A quick Google search showed me a price of $134.48 "with free discount" at Walmart's pharmacy. That's for 30 tablets of 0.6mg *generic Colchicine*. Gee, what a bargain! I always buy my generic poison at WalMart, they have all the best deals!

There are plenty of non-toxic options for gout that are very *affordable*, which you will see below, so what's the point in quite literally feeding people *poison*, calling it "medicine" and then ripping them off on the price to boot? If anyone can give me a good answer to that question I'd be interested in hearing it. As far as I'm concerned the use of this toxic poison as "medicine" is totally unnecessary and the price...well, let me just say that it's organized crime, the "legal" kind, with the blessing of the federal government for the drug companies to sodomize the common people.

Now I'd like to address the other drug commonly prescribed for gout, *Allopurinol*, the one that I took on and off for years until I discovered that I can control gout symptoms naturally. Are you ready? Ok here goes.

RxList.com states:

"Some serious side effects of Zyloprim (Allopurinol) may include swelling of mouth and lips, severe skin rashes, infections, eye irritation, hepatitis, appetite and weight loss, and painful or bloody urination. Zyloprim should be used during pregnancy only if clearly needed and used with caution in women who are breastfeeding; benefits vs. harm to the fetus or infant should be considered."

"Stop using allopurinol and call your doctor at once if you have a serious side effect such as:

- fever, sore throat, and headache with a severe blistering, peeling, and red skin rash;
- the first sign of any skin rash, no matter how mild;
- pain or bleeding when you urinate;
- nausea, upper stomach pain, itching, loss of appetite, weight loss, dark urine, clay-

colored stools
- jaundice (yellowing of the skin or eyes);
- urinating less than usual or not at all;
- joint pain, flu symptoms;
- severe tingling, numbness, pain, muscle weakness; or
- easy bruising, unusual bleeding (nose, mouth, vagina, or rectum), purple or red pinpoint spots under your skin.

Less serious side effects may include:

- vomiting, diarrhea;
- drowsiness, headache;
- changes in your sense of taste; or
- muscle pain."

Full article is here: *http://www.rxlist.com/zyloprim-side-effects-drug-center.htm*

And again from *PubMed.gov*:

"A life-threatening toxicity syndrome consisting of an erythematous, desquamative skin rash, fever, hepatitis, eosinophilia, and worsening renal function in 78 patients receiving allopurinol is described. In a majority of cases, the development of this syndrome was associated with the use of standard (200 to 400 mg per day) doses of allopurinol in patients with renal insufficiency."

Full article is here: *http://www.ncbi.nlm.nih.gov/pubmed/6691361*

Wow. OK. So *both* drugs are potentially *deadly*. Nice "medicine"! *Again*, is there any good reason why these drugs should be used when safe, natural and effective treatments exist? The fact that "doctors" ignore the safe and natural treatments (that I am about to list below), and prescribe *poison* to people instead simply makes my blood boil. That's health care? Not in my view. No sane person can consider that health care. It's not. It's a crime against humanity. Even if only a single person died from these drugs, it was *absolutely unnecessary,* because these drugs are absolutely unnecessary!

And the price on *Allopurinol* at WalMart's bargain pharmacy? $4.00. Not so bad. It's nice to know that I can purchase potentially deadly poison at such a remarkable price!

Now let's get started with the information that all people who suffer from gout attacks need to know. This is how to control your gout symptoms safely and naturally with no "doctor" visits, no pharmacy and no deadly poisons, and without getting sodomized or having your money stolen from you by drug companies.

When I learned of the toxic side effects of *Allopurinol* I quickly stopped taking the drug. I then began scouring the internet for other options. I quickly discovered that the key to avoiding gout attacks and flair-ups is to maintain a balanced pH. I saw a *YouTube.com* video commercial for a coral calcium product. It was a man stirring the calcium into glasses of red colored water, a very acidic color. After he stirred the calcium into the water the color changed to purple, indicating strong alkaline. He then said "This is the key to avoiding gout attacks, neutralizing acid and maintaining an alkaline state. Use this product and you'll never have gout again."

Balancing your body's pH is kind of tricky depending upon your lifestyle, but the idea is to keep a proper ratio of acidity to alkalinity in your bodily fluids. To test your pH you can purchase pH test strips at any health food store. The most common tests are urine and saliva. Opinions vary on "optimal pH values" for urine and saliva, some sources go as low as 6 and others say it's as high as 7, but despite anyone's difference in opinion, a neutral (balanced) pH is 7. You'll see that when you buy your test strips. 7 is a perfect balance, therefore that is what you are shooting for. Gout is caused by the build up of acid in the blood stream, uric acid in particular, therefore if you can keep your pH up around the 6 or 7 marker you'll likely never have to worry about gout ever again.

One of the main causes of my gout problems was consumption of soda pop, which is very acidic, very high in uric acid content which caused me to have an acidic pH for most of my life. When I started seeking natural solutions for gout and learned about pH balance I was basically addicted to diet soda, and had not yet made it to the point in my life where I was ready to quit, but I did use the coral calcium and it did a good job of offsetting the acidity of the soda. I still felt "gouty" from time to time, but I never had major attacks anymore. Coral calcium is a very good, if not the best, way to raise the body's pH. Alkaline water from the health food store works very well also. The higher the pH of the water, the better. A teaspoon of baking soda in an 8-ounce glass of water will raise your pH real nicely too. Make sure it's a high quality brand like *Arm & Hammer* or one that specifically states that it's *aluminum free*. **Very important**, as many brands of baking soda *do contain* aluminum! Do not exceed two teaspoons per day, preferably in separate doses, and don't take it long term, a few weeks at a time maximum.

So, how's *this* for a medicine? Cherries! Yes, *Tart Cherry Extract*, or just eating cherries every day, will ease gout symptoms. It was once an unproven "folk remedy" but now it is backed by genuine science. *PubMed.com* listed a study on their website that was published online on September 28th, 2012 which states:

> "Our study included 633 individuals with gout. Cherry intake over a 2-day period was associated with a 35% lower risk of gout attacks compared with no intake...The effect of cherry intake persisted across subgroups stratified by sex, obesity status, purine intake, alcohol use, diuretic use, and use of antigout medications...These findings suggest that cherry intake is associated with a lower risk of gout attacks."

> **Full article here**: *http://www.ncbi.nlm.nih.gov/pubmed/23023818*

I found a great article online, with all sources cited, and I'd like to share some of it with you here. This is from the *Life Extension Magazine* website at *lef.org* and the article is entitled *"The Anti-Inflammatory Properties of Tart Cherry"*:

> "On October 17, 2005, the FDA sent out warning letters to cherry growers insisting that they cease making substantiated health claims that specific chemicals found in cherries could reduce pain and inflammation.

> The FDA wanted cherry growers to stop citing published scientific studies showing that cherries are packed with unique anthocyanins and other compounds that naturally mediate the inflammatory process. These compounds deliver comparable anti-inflammatory activity to ibuprofen (Advil®) and naproxen (Aleve®)—but without the significant side effects!

> Standard treatment for muscle pain and inflammation has been with nonsteroidal anti-inflammatory drugs. With over 111 million prescriptions and accounting for around 60% of over-the-counter pain reliever sales in the USA alone, these are some of the most commonly used types of medications. But because they can have deadly side effects, including gastric bleeding, heart attack, and kidney failure, the search for natural agents that could prove more beneficial and safer has gained increased attention.

> The compounds found in cherries modulate numerous pathways to protect against other conditions associated with inflammation—including cancer, cardiovascular disease, metabolic syndrome, and Alzheimer's disease. For example, tart cherry constituents can switch critical genes off and on; modulate cell-signaling molecules like tumor necrosis factor; and target multiple cardiovascular factors—producing, in one study model, an astounding 65% reduction in early mortality!

> In this article, you will learn of the multiple benefits found in cherries that the FDA did not want to be publicized."

> **Full article is here:** *http://www.lef.org/Magazine/2013/6/Anti-Inflammatory-Properties-of-Tart-Cherry/Page-01*

Gee whiz Wally, I wonder why the FDA didn't want that information publicized? Could it be because drug profits come first and human health comes last? You tell me.

I personally have used *Coral Calcium* and *Tart Cherry Extract* for years, in combination with *Celery Seed Extract* (which also neutralizes acid and has anti-inflammatory properties), *Bromelain* and *Turmeric* (which have anti-inflammatory properties) and never had a gout attack, not one, even though I was still drinking my acidic diet soda every day by the gallon. I hate to admit how destructive I was being to myself, but the diet soda was pretty much all I ever drank. It was my only liquid intake, for the most part. I'm only telling you this to illustrate my point concerning these supplements; if they will work to cure gout on a man who was abusing himself with diet soda to such an extreme then I'd say it's safe to assume that these supplements would work on just about anybody! If you have gout then you have absolutely nothing to lose by giving these great alternatives to poisonous and expensive drugs a shot! Remember, always inquire with your primary care provider before starting any new treatments.

Something else that I have to mention is that diet soda contains a toxic poison called *aspartame* (not to mention that it's loaded up with chemicals). Aspartame is associate with over 92 different health problems, including depression and seizures. By stopping aspartame consumption I eliminated a very toxic substance from my diet. Aspartame is an ingredient in *thousands* of "sugar free" products. Do yourself a favor and stop consuming it! For more information on aspartame see ***Appendix C***.

During my ongoing studies on herbalism and natural medicine, I have learned that there are many other supplements that are effective for painful arthritis conditions, including Osteoarthritis and Rheumatoid Arthritis:

- Boron
- Boswellia
- Cat's Claw Extract
- Chondroitin
- Devil's Claw Extract
- Fish Collagen
- Fish Oils
- Glucosamine (this one assisted my knees in growing new cartilage! They were nearly bone on bone and very painful. My knee problems vanished within a few months of starting on this!)
- MSM
- SAM-e
- Stinging Nettles
- Turmeric
- White Willow Bark Extract (contains salicin, the main ingredient in aspirin)

If you suffer from any form of arthritis or knee problems, these safe and natural supplements will be of great benefit to you. For various forms of arthritis "doctors" will often provide dangerous anti-inflammatory drugs and narcotic pain medicines that are physically addictive such as *Oxycodone* and others. In other words, as I've said again and again in this book, "doctors" don't look for the *root cause* of things, they simply pull out a prescription pad and offer up a drug instead, which, again, isn't health care, and is an act in criminal negligence. Trust me on this one, you'd be *much* better off going the safe and natural route with a combination of these supplements and herbs. Call me crazy, but I think that's a bit more logical. It's your body, so by all means, do what you wish, but when the truth stares you in the face, the best advice would be to *take heed*.

Type 2 Diabetes

Considering how much you know about my health history by now, it should come as no surprise to you that I was diagnosed with type 2 diabetes at the age of 34. I certainly was diabetic long before that, but I didn't see "doctors" much, and I had to be hospitalized before I was officially diagnosed.

I woke up one morning with a terrible pain in my chest area. I thought that I might have been having a heart attack, and so I called Mom and asked her to give me a ride to the emergency room. They took a few blood samples and some x-rays and came back to tell me that my blood sugar level was sky high at over 600 and that my pancreas was severely inflamed. I was immediately sent to their luxury suite known as ICU or *Intensive Care Unit* where I enjoyed a ten day stay receiving a disgusting looking green slime through a tube for nourishment. My official diagnosis was "acute pancreatitus". I wasn't allowed to eat or drink for more than a week because they said that they wanted the pancreas to rest and heal.

During the course of my ten day stay my gout problem decided to pop up and say hello. My feet were swollen to nearly twice their normal size. To my amazement and disgust, the "doctor" in charge of my care flat out *refused* to give me any form of medication for my feet. I was asking for an anti-inflammatory, and her reply was "No. Your pancreas needs to rest." When I asked about an intravenous shot she kept saying "no" for a reason that was totally unclear. She had no logical reason to refuse a liquid drug in shot form, but she kept saying "no". I was in no mood for any bullshit, so I fired her and they had to send in another "doctor" to take over my care. When I told him what the problem was he kind of smirked, indicating that he thought my first "doctor" wasn't too bright, and then said something like "Well, there are liquid anti-inflammatory drugs that can be given in shot form, which eliminates the need to over-work the pancreas." Simple solution! He immediately ordered the nurses to start giving me regular shots and within a couple of days my feet were nearly back to normal. Thinking back on that, I still find it amazing that my first "doctor" was that amazingly stupid. The one that replaced her resolved the problem in about five seconds. Quick and easy! After I was released I received a letter in the mail from the first "doctor" telling me that I wasn't allowed to be her patient ever again, as if I was was somehow interested in that possibility? I fired you, remember!?

Something else that I found amazing and disgusting during my stay was that the hospital sent in a physical therapist to try and get me to *walk* on my swollen feet! I wasn't in my best spirits during this ordeal and my patience was very short. She was pushy, so I told that person to "take a hike" and she left clearly shook up. What were they thinking, asking a man with severely painful gout inflamed feet to walk? Have they no knowledge of how severely painful gout is? These are health care professionals? Not even close, thank you very much. Idiots would be a better description.

Before I was released I was given clear instructions on diet, a glucose meter with instructions on how to test my blood sugar, and of course, I was given a prescription for very expensive insulin. I followed their advice for a few months until I discovered that their methods are an act in criminal negligence, and then I began treating myself.

Let's review a standard breakfast for diabetics as recommended by the *American Diabetes Association*. This was the basic meal plan that I was on:

"6 oz. Orange Juice, a bowl of plain oatmeal, two slices of toast, decaf coffee or tea with 1 tsp of sugar."

Ok; let's start with orange juice. Orange juice is *extremely* high in natural sugars. One cup contains 29.5 grams of carbohydrates and only .25 grams come from fiber. Fiber carbs don't impact blood sugar, so they "don't count", but the remaining 29.25 grams of carbs will turn into pure glucose (*sugar!*) in the body after consumption. Not a good choice for a diabetic!

Now oatmeal; one cup contains 27 grams of carbs and only 4 come from fiber. Keeping in mind that carbs turn into pure glucose (*sugar!*) in the body after consumption, the rest is just like eating pure *sugar!*

Now "toast" or sliced bread: One slice of white bread has 36 grams of carbs and only 1.5 of those come from fiber. The rest of them impact blood sugar because they turn into glucose (*sugar!*).

Something that I learned while reading the book *Wheat Belly* by Dr. William Davis is that eating two slices of wheat bread is actually *worse than eating a Snickers bar!* As I mentioned in the introduction, the glycemic index rating for pure sugar is only 59, while the GI rating for wheat bread is 72! White bread is rated at 70. A Snickers bar only rates at 41!

After reviewing the dietary recommendations for diabetics from the *American Diabetes Association* and the scientific facts that I've just outlined concerning that meal plan, anyone with an IQ above 12 should be able to tell me what the problem is! Remember, this is *just breakfast*. For anyone who doesn't know anything about nutrition this might look like a pretty healthy meal plan. But it's *not*. Far from it. *Especially for a diabetic patient!*

Overall, we have a "diabetic meal plan" that is dominated by *sugar!* This plan contains over 150 grams of carbs, and it's just a light breakfast! Never mind lunch and dinner! As a diabetic, if I were to eat a meal like this breakfast example my blood sugar levels would *skyrocket*. And that's precisely what happened when I followed their bullshit advice.

The vast majority of type 2 diabetic patients, including myself, do in fact have a pancreas that produces insulin just fine, it's just that our cells have become *insulin resistant*, which is why we've become diabetic. The standard American diet (S.A.D.) is loaded with carbs, and when you eat nothing but carbs your pancreas basically panics and starts producing massive insulin on overdrive. Because of the overload of insulin your cells soon become insulin resistant. The insulin will try to deliver the glucose to the cells, but the cells will say "No. I've had enough! Go away!" and then you're stuck with a bunch of excess glucose *and* insulin floating around in your blood stream! And that is why we have a diabetes epidemic in this country. With drinks like *Coca-Cola* which contain 9 ½ teaspoons of sugar per 12 ounce can being a main staple in the standard American diet, and with the USDA putting carbohydrates and "healthy whole grains" which turn into pure sugar on the bottom of their food pyramid (see introduction), is there any wonder why people are turning diabetic? It doesn't take a rocket scientist to figure it out! They are **insulin resistant**! The vast majority of them!

As a diabetes type 2 patient, I can say that it didn't matter how many of their insulin shots I took, my blood sugar was always high, and that's because I was insulin resistant, just like the vast majority of type 2 patients!

Which brings us to *yet more incompetence* from the *American Diabetes Association.* First, they pump diabetics full of sugar by recommending a diet plan that is high in carbohydrates, and then they say "Here you go, here's some expensive insulin for you!" (which makes nice profits for the drugs companies but it certainly doesn't help the diabetic patient). Insulin doesn't work on people who are insulin resistant! Why would you want to give insulin to someone who is insulin resistant? That's kind of like giving a pair of gloves to a man with no hands! It might be a workable solution for the type 1 patient, because they aren't insulin resistant and their pancreas doesn't produce insulin, but the majority of diabetes patients including myself are type 2 patients with *insulin resistance.* Their diet plan and their insulin simply didn't work for me! It did me far more harm than good, as a matter of fact *it did me nothing but harm.* I was eating lots of carbs (sugars) *because they told me to* and I was shooting up their insulin three times a day *because they told me to* but my body's cells refused to accept the insulin and of course my blood sugar levels remained elevated! I was being slowly and systematically *killed* by so-called "medical professionals" and that's no exaggeration *that's the plain truth* of the matter. They were in fact *killing me* with their so-called "care" and that's what they continue to do to this very day with millions of people who are type 2 diabetics! Fortunately for me, I was intelligent enough to figure it out. *Many people, probably most people, are not.*

When I figured out that mainstream "medicine" was quite literally killing me it didn't take me long to find a solution. My Dad had informed me on low carbohydrate diets and he had said to me in a factual tone of voice "I know you'll be on this diet someday son". I also had an Aunt that was a firm advocate of the low carb lifestyle and she had informed me of the numerous health benefits. It didn't make any sense to me that a person with diabetes should be loading up their diet with carbohydrates and *sugar*(!), so I started my research on the subject. I started with the book *Dr. Atkin's New Diet Revolution* by the controversial maverick (and hero), Dr. Robert C. Atkins, M.D. I read the book from cover to cover in a matter of days. When I got to the part about diabetes a big light went off in my head. "I'm trying this!" I thought. And I did.

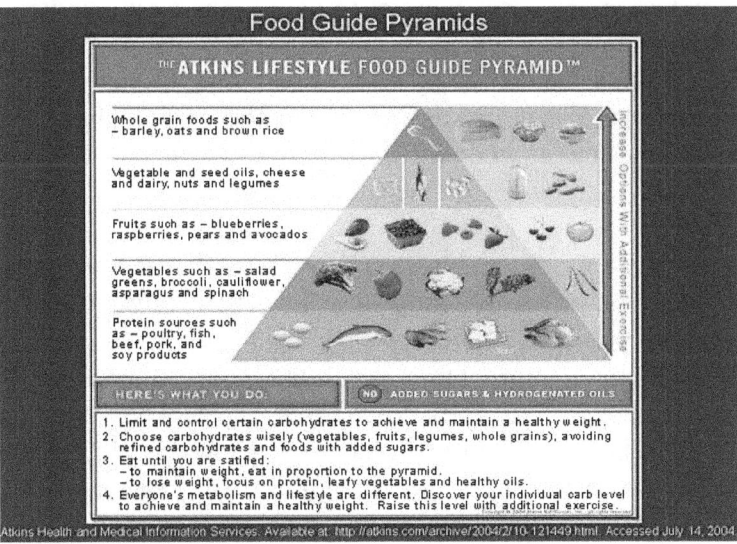

As you can see, the Atkins lifestyle food pyramid is much different than the USDA's (see introduction). Note that it marginalizes those so-called "healthy whole grains" and basically makes them taboo, only to be used *minimally* (because they're all *sugar*!). And note that the bottom of the pyramid is based upon proteins and non-starchy vegetables.

I started eating burgers and salads, green vegetables, chicken, fish and other low carb foods (it's not necessary to eat red meats if you don't want to while you're on a low carb diet, there are plenty of other options). I ate a maximum of 20 grams of carbs per day. I followed the Atkins food pyramid exactly and within 24 hours I started seeing my blood sugar levels taking a nose dive. Gradually, within a couple of weeks, my blood sugar completely stabilized and I was no longer using insulin. My blood sugar readings were consistently in the normal range for healthy, non-diabetic people. It got to the point where checking my blood sugar was a waste of a perfectly good test strip, because I had successfully "cured" myself of diabetes. As long as I stayed on a low carb lifestyle, my diabetes didn't exist, it remained in a state of hibernation.

I did some experimenting with carbohydrate levels. I tried eating a 100 gram (of carbs) pizza to see what it did to my blood sugar and quickly learned that 100 grams was far too much. I came to know how many carbohydrates my body can handle without spiking my blood sugar through trial and error. It turned out that I cannot eat more than about 30 grams per sitting, but that's ok because even if you aren't diabetic sugars and carbohydrates, especially the refined and processed flours and things like that, are terrible for health in general. *All* people are better off avoiding those things.

When I figure out just how effective a diet low in carbohydrates was on my blood sugar levels and how excellent it worked for controlling my diabetes, I was happy that I found a solution, of course, but I was also extremely pissed off. I was very upset with "doctors" and all I could think is "They never told me about this! They call themselves 'doctors' but never told me about this! They had me shoot insulin three times a day and eat carbs instead! *&$#@*!!!" That was the beginning of my disillusionment with "doctors". From that point forward I no longer trusted them and I questioned everything they said. If they couldn't give me the simple truth about a life threatening disease called diabetes then I couldn't trust them any longer. Not a chance! No way! It was then that I realized that I'd have to start doing my own research and accepting responsibility for my own health, because I knew that "doctors" were worthless.

At one point I fell off of the low carb bandwagon and started eating things that I shouldn't have been eating. As a result, my blood sugar was no longer under control. At that point I tried an oral drug called *Metformin*. I was on it for only a short time when I started having bladder problems such as urgency to urinate, blood in my urine and lack of bladder control. I couldn't for the life of me figure out what was causing it until my aunt, who was a nurse all of her life, casually told me that diabetes medications are known to cause bladder cancer and other issues. At that point a big light went off in my head. Ah ha! And, of course, when I stopped taking Metformin the bladder infection went away almost immediately.

When I went in to see the "doctor" I told her that I'd stopped the *Metformin* due to bladder infection. She got right up in my face and treated me like a child, scolding me and telling me that if I didn't keep taking that drug she'd never have me as a patient ever again. I tried to make it clear to her that the bladder infection cleared up *only because I had stopped taking Metformin* and she denied that it could have that effect. She also tried to tell me that *Metformin* "protects against bladder cancer". My reply was "that's debatable" and she stormed out of the room and sent in a messenger to inform me that I was no longer her patient. I wrote her a letter several months later after doing some research and I'd like to share some excerpts here:

"You said that Metformin could never possibly cause a bladder infection. I shared my experience of the drug with you, because I thought maybe you'd be willing to listen to what I had to say. I told you that as soon as I stopped taking Metformin the bladder infection suddenly went away. Gee, what an odd coincidence. Start the drug; bladder infection. Stop the drug; bladder infection goes away. Interesting indeed. I'm not a rocket scientist, but I think I see a correlation there. Of course, listening was nothing you were interested in doing. You were only interested in defending your miracle drug. If you bother to do even a little bit of research on the subject of Metformin and bladder infections you'll quickly see that I'm not the only person who has ever experienced that problem:

eHealthMe.com states:

"Bladder infection is found among people who take Metformin, especially for people who are female, 60+ old, have been taking the drug for 1 - 6 months, also take medication Metformin hcl, and have Diabetes. We study 97,426 people who have side effects while taking Metformin from FDA and social media. Among them, 1,631 have Bladder infection. Find out below who they are, when they have Bladder infection and more." - *http://www.ehealthme.com/ds/metformin/bladder+infection*

DoubleCheckMD.com states:

"GlipiZIDE-metformin may cause urinary tract infection. This drug may also cause the following symptoms that are related to urinary tract infection: Burning with urination, Discomfort with urination." - *http://doublecheckmd.com/EffectsDetail.do? dname=glipiZIDE-metformin&sid=45353&eid=3113*

Let's take a look at Drugs.com:

"In addition to its needed effects, some unwanted effects may be caused by metformin / saxagliptin: Anxiety, bladder pain, bloody or cloudy urine...." - *http://www.drugs.com/sfx/metformin-saxagliptin-side-effects.html*

I'll not drone on. I've made my point. You were wrong. Metformin can and does cause bladder infections. Case closed. Now let's look at the next thing you said.

You said that Metformin "protects against bladder cancer."

OK, so I've already proven that it causes bladder infections, and if it causes bladder infections I'd say that it's a very safe bet that it doesn't "protect against bladder cancer." And that's exactly what a recent study from Feb. 2014 showed:

"No Bladder-Cancer Protection With Metformin, New Study Finds":
http://www.medscape.com/viewarticle/820378

And from the University of Oxford in August of 2012:

"Research published online this month led by researchers at the University of Oxford, including DTU, suggests that the diabetes drug metformin does not prevent people from developing cancer. The study, funded by Diabetes UK and published in the journal Diabetologia, analyzed the largest collection of clinical trials data ever used to study metformin and cancer. The researchers examined data from nine randomized controlled trials (RCTs) published in the scientific literature. The trials had tested metformin alongside placebo, usual care or other treatments for diabetes in more than 11,500 people without pre-existing cancer, and on average, followed-up the patients after they had completed the trial for four years." - *https://www.dtu.ox.ac.uk/generic/article.php?213*

So, no. Metformin doesn't protect against cancer and yes, it causes bladder infections. Not to mention, what sane person wants to take a drug with a list of side effects like this? - "Abdominal or stomach discomfort, cough or hoarseness, decreased appetite, diarrhea, fast or shallow breathing, fever or chills, general feeling of discomfort, lower back or side pain, muscle pain or cramping, painful or difficult urination, sleepiness, Anxiety, blurred vision, chest discomfort, cold sweats, coma, confusion, cool, pale skin, depression, difficult or labored breathing, dizziness, fast, irregular, pounding, or racing heartbeat or pulse, feeling of warmth, headache, increased hunger, increased sweating, nausea, nervousness, nightmares, redness of the face, neck, arms, and occasionally, upper chest, seizures, shakiness, shortness of breath, slurred speech, tightness in the chest, unusual tiredness or weakness, wheezing, Behavior change similar to being drunk, difficulty with concentrating, drowsiness, lack or loss of strength, restless sleep, unusual sleepiness" - *http://www.drugs.com/sfx/metformin-side-effects.html*

Whew!! And just think; you stormed out of the office and refused to have anything to do with me ever again because I refused to take this drug!! Metformin might lower blood sugar, but that's one hell of a trade off!!"

I never did hear anything back from that "doctor" and that experience was just another nail in the coffin as far as I was concerned. I was determined to liberate myself from "doctors" once and for all. I was fed up and wasn't going to put up with it any more. Obviously, a thinking person isn't allowed to think, we're all just supposed to nod our heads in agreement with everything the "doctor" says, and obey their commands for us to take various drugs with long lists of side effects, we're not supposed to research one bit, and if we ask questions then we're immediately marginalized and made out to be trouble makers. That's called using bully tactics, and that's called sheer arrogance. Pardon me, but I believe in doing research on substances that I'm told are supposed to be good for me so that I can verify that it is, in fact, going to make me healthier. I like to know the pros and cons, I like to know what the side effects are, I like to measure benefits vs. possible harm done when it comes to things that I put into **my body** and if any "doctor" that I happen to be seeing has any problem with that whatsoever then they can piss off, plain and simple.

As far as herbs and supplements go, there are many that assist in lowering and controlling blood sugar levels and they are actually proven to be far more effective than drugs. Taking toxins like *Metformin* is totally and completely unnecessary:

- Bitter Melon (Bergamot)
- Cinnamon
- Essiac (also known as "Ojibwa")
- Fenugreek
- Garcinia Cambogia (Hydroxycitric acid)
- Ginseng
- Grape Seed Extract (Resveratrol)
- Gymnema Sylvester
- Milk Thistle
- Mulberry Extract
- Pine Bark Extract (Pycnogenol)
- Psyllium Husks (or fiber supplements)
- Sage
- Touchi Extract

I personally take *Gymnema Sylvester* just for good measure, I also take *Resveratrol* for cancer prevention (more on that later), and milk thistle for liver cleansing (more on that later too), but ultimately, I use a low carb lifestyle to control my blood sugar. Using diet is by far the most effective method. Benefits of the low carb lifestyle include blood sugar level control, insulin level control, lowered blood pressure, lowered triglycerides and cholesterol, appetite control, more energy, plus much more. *There is no dietary lifestyle that is healthier than the low carbohydrate lifestyle*, and I shall prove that to you in the upcoming chapters.

Hypertension (High Blood Pressure)

I mentioned earlier that the standard American diet (S.A.D.) is loaded with sugars and carbohydrates, which causes blood sugar levels to rise, which causes insulin levels to rise, which causes the cells to become resistant to insulin, which causes an excess of glucose (blood sugar) and insulin to be floating around in the blood stream, and of course, it also makes triglycerides skyrocket! When the blood stream is loaded up with excess glucose and insulin, not to mention triglycerides, what happens? It *thickens the blood*, which in turn *causes blood pressure to rise*, which is why people with diabetes very commonly have high blood pressure. I was no exception. At one point my blood pressure was nearly 150/105 which is dangerously high.

Blood pressure readings are calculated by measuring the amount of pressure on the walls of the arteries. The top number, the "systolic", measures the amount of pressure while the heart is pumping. The bottom number, the "diastolic", measures the amount of pressure in between beats while the heart is at rest. Considering that 120/80 is considered the standard average, my blood pressure was very out of whack. I definitely had something to be concerned about.

I was discussing the health benefits of a low carb diet in the last section. Concerning blood pressure, when you go on a low carb diet you're basically eliminating all sugar (carbs are sugars!) from your diet. When you stop the sugars obviously your blood glucose level is going to go down (which is why it is so effective for diabetes). When your glucose goes down, obviously your insulin levels are going to go down, and your triglycerides will go down as well. As a result of having less glucose, less insulin and less triglycerides floating around in your bloodstream, your blood is *thinner*, and guess what happens? It causes *blood pressure to go down* of course! And that's precisely what happened to me when I started on a low carb diet.

When my blood pressure was high "doctors" had me on a drug called *Lisinopril* also known as *Prinivil*. I'd like to address this drug before moving on.

Drugs.com states:

> "Lisinopril side effects
>
> Call your doctor at once if you have:
>
> - a light-headed feeling, like you might pass out;
> - little or no urinating;
> - swelling, rapid weight gain;
> - fever, chills, body aches, flu symptoms;
> - tired feeling, muscle weakness, and pounding or uneven heartbeats;
> - psoriasis (raised, silvery flaking of the skin);
> - chest pain; or
> - high potassium (slow heart rate, weak pulse, muscle weakness, tingly feeling);
>
> Common lisinopril side effects may include:
>
> - cough;
> - dizziness, drowsiness, headache;
> - depressed mood;
> - nausea, vomiting, diarrhea, upset stomach; or
> - mild skin itching or rash.
>
> This is not a complete list of side effects and others may occur."

Full article is here: _http://www.drugs.com/lisinopril.html_

WebMD.com gives the same list of standard side effects, plus the following:

> "This drug may rarely cause serious (possibly fatal) liver problems. Tell your doctor right away if you notice any of the following rare but serious side effects: yellowing eyes/skin, dark urine, severe stomach/abdominal pain, persistent nausea/vomiting."

Full article is here: _http://www.webmd.com/drugs/2/drug-6873/lisinopril-oral/details_

And so once again, a drug that I was prescribed by "doctors" turns out to be potentially _deadly_ ("possibly fatal") and even if it wasn't potentially deadly the list of side effects is clearly undesirable. "Doctors" told me _nothing_ of natural ways to lower blood pressure, they told me _nothing_ of relaxation/stress reduction techniques, they told me _nothing_ about natural dietary supplements that lower blood pressure. To their credit they _did_ mention getting more exercise and drinking more water. But this drug is dangerous, as are _all_ blood pressure lowering drugs, and again their use is totally and completely _unnecessary_ (except in cases of emergency). I don't oppose drugs in emergency situations and sometimes, because these blood pressure lowering drugs can be more powerful than herbs and supplements, they can be useful for emergencies. In cases like that, where its the last resort, by all means, use the drugs, but in 95% of cases that simply isn't the case! And look at how many blood pressure lowering drugs they're selling and how much money they're making every year! *$$ Billions!! $$*

In the *WebMD.com* article quoted above they also say this:

> "Lisinopril is an ACE inhibitor and works by relaxing blood vessels so that blood can flow more easily."

OK. Fine. But if I'm *dead* from the treatment how well will my blood be flowing *then*? Considering the fact that there are safe, natural and side effect free ACE Inhibitors that are readily available, I'd say that the promotion of this drug onto innocent, ignorant and unsuspecting people is a crime against humanity. Most people trust doctors, and taking advantage of that trust by giving them potentially deadly drugs is criminal negligence and it certainly isn't health care. If even one person has died as a result of this drug, then it was totally unnecessary!

So, do you know anyone taking blood thinners? Sounds innocent enough, right? Well check out this article from *NaturalNews.com* entitled *"Doctors Give **Rat Poison** to Heart Patients for Fifty Years"*:

> "A Bloomberg report just told us that millions of people worldwide have been taking **rat poison** as a prescription blood thinner. It also said that the risk of bleeding in the brain with this drug called warfarin was one of the drug's most feared complications."
>
> **Full article is here**: *http://www.naturalnews.com/026960_poison_patients _doctors.html#ixzz3YHG4z8Vf*

So who thought of that idea? Who in their right mind would consider using *rat poison* as "medicine"? Certainly not me! I have three words concerning that; *what the fuck?* The good news is that you don't have to take rat poison! Natural blood thinners (anticoagulants) are listed below!

The following is quoted from an article entitled *"Evaluation of Nutritional Support with Bonito Peptides in Patients with Hypertension: Summary of Clinical Experience"* which details the clinical results of bonito fish peptides for people with high blood pressure. (A *Google.com* search for the article will bring up many links to the .pdf file so that you can read the whole thing):

"The results of these case studies suggest that bonito peptides are approximately 64% effective in reducing BP in borderline and mildly hypertensive subjects. In these short - term clinical trials, no serious adverse effects were reported, suggesting that bonito peptides have an excellent safety profile."

And that's just one of many examples of natural ACE Inhibitors. Others include oligomeric proanthocyanidins (OPCs) which can be found in hundreds of different plants but are highly concentrated in *Pine Bark Extract*, *Grape Seed Extract* and *Hawthorn Berries*. Citrus bioflavonoids can be found in numerous fruits and also have a very powerful blood pressure (and cholesterol) lowering effect. More on cholesterol in the next section.

I have researched blood pressure lowering supplements extensively due to my own bouts with high blood pressure, and unless you're at an emergency high level, there is **absolutely no need to take drugs for high blood pressure, ever**.

[**Very important**: *If you decide to go off of your blood pressure lowering drug(s) only do so slowly and gradually and under the supervision of your primary care provider. Stopping suddenly with blood pressure meds can be very dangerous and can cause heart attacks and strokes!*]

Safe and natural, side-effect free supplements that lower blood pressure include:

- Ashwaganda
- Bonito Fish Peptides
- Burdock Root
- Cayenne Pepper (anticoagulant)
- Celery Seed Extract (or 4 oz per day raw celery, anticoagulant)
- Chicory
- Citrus bioflavonoids
- Coleus Forskohlii (*may interact with blood thinning drugs*)
- Curry Powder (anticoagulant)
- Dandelion (natural diuretic)
- Ginkgo Biloba (promotes blood circulation to the brain)
- Golden Rod
- Grape Seed Extract (anticoagulant)
- Hawthorn (simply one of the best herbs for heart health)
- Hibiscus
- L-Arginine (promotes blood flow and circulation)
- Linden Flower
- Nattokinase (powerful enzyme anticoagulant, breaks down blood clots)
- Olive Leaf (*may interact with blood thinning drugs*)
- Oregano (anticoagulant)
- Parsley (natural diuretic)
- Pine Bark
- Potassium (this has to be in balance with sodium levels!)
- Quercitan
- Thyme (anticoagulant)
- Turmeric (anticoagulant)
- White Willow Bark (this is what aspirin is made out of, anticoagulant)

And that's not a full list. Quite frankly, there are too many to list, but I listed the best ones for this particular condition. Garlic does the trick too, but I ***don't recommend*** garlic. Garlic is a very useful herb, one of the best, it thins blood, lowers blood pressure, lowers cholesterol, boosts immunity, fights colds and infections, fights cancer, cleanses blood and much more. But, unfortunately, *unless it's absolutely necessary* I don't recommend you use garlic, at all, period. Garlic is proven to desynchronize the two hemispheres of the brain, cloud thinking, slow down reaction time and more:

> "The reason garlic is so toxic, the sulphone hydroxyl ion penetrates the blood brain barrier, just like DMSO, and is a specific poison for higher life forms and brain cells. We discovered this much to our horror, when I was the world's largest manufacturer of ethical EEG biofeedback equipment. We'd have people come back from lunch that looked clinically dead on the encephalograph, which we used to calibrate their progress. 'Well, what happened?' 'Well, I went to an Italian restaurant and there was some garlic in my salad dressing!'
>
> So we had 'em sign things that they won't touch garlic before classes or we were wasting their time, and money and my time. I guess those of you who are pilots or have been in flight tests... I was in flight test engineering in Doc Hallan's group in the 1950's. The flight surgeon would come around every month and remind all of us: 'Don't you dare touch any garlic 72 hours before you fly one of our airplanes, because it'll double or triple your reaction time. You're three times slower than you would be if you'd [not] had a few drops of garlic.'
>
> Well, we didn't know why for 20 years, until I owned the Alpha-Metrics Corporation. We were building biofeedback equipment and found out that garlic totally desynchronizes your brain waves. So I funded a study at Stanford and, sure enough, they found that it's a poison. You can rub a clove of garlic on your foot - on the sole of your foot - and you can smell it shortly later on your wrists. So it penetrates the body. This is why DMSO smells a lot like garlic: that sulphone hydroxyl ion penetrates all the barriers including the corpus callosum in the brain. Any of you who are organic gardeners know that if you don't want to use DDT, garlic will kill anything in the way of insects. Now, most people have heard most of their lives that garlic is good for you, and we put those people in the same class of ignorance as the mothers who at the turn of the century would buy morphine sulphate in the drugstore and give it to their babies to put 'em to sleep. If you have any patients who have low-grade headaches or attention deficit [disorder], they can't quite focus on the computer in the afternoon, just do an experiment - you owe it to yourselves. Take those people off garlic and see how much better they get, very,very shortly. And then let them eat a little garlic after about three weeks. They'll say: 'My God, I had no idea that this was the cause of our problems.' And this includes the de-skunked garlic's, Kyolic, some of the other products. Very unpopular, but I've got to tell you the truth."
>
> - Dr Robert C. Beck, DSc., lecture at the *Whole Life Expo*, Seattle, WA, USA, 1996

In other words, avoid garlic! (Yes, I know, it is so good on bread though!)

As an herbalist, I created my own ten herb blood pressure blend and made it into a tincture that I take three times daily. The ingredients are one part each of *Olive Leaf, Hawthorne Berries,*

Ashwaganda, Golden Rod, Dandelion Root, Hibiscus, Linden Flowers, Celery Seed, Gingko Biloba and *Burdock Root.* And yes, it works for me better than *Lisinopril,* thank you very much. My blood pressure is now 126/76 at time of writing. Just say no to drugs!

[*As an update to the second addition nearly ten months later, I have weaned myself off of the blood pressure tincture, and am now taking far less natural medicine for my condition, less than half as much I'd say, and my blood pressure is consistently stable at around 120/80, in other words, the initial herbal treatment combined with my diet and exercise routine corrected the majority of the root cause of the problem, eliminating the need to continue with such a heavy dose of blood pressure lowering herbs.*]

Hyperlipidemia (High Cholesterol/Triglycerides)

Cholesterol, the great villain that causes heart disease. Supposedly. "Keep your cholesterol low!" they say, "or you'll die soon!" It's that old scare them into submission tactic. After all, statin drugs just happen to be the biggest selling pharmaceutical drug in the history of mainstream medicine, and that's a fact. Statin drugs like *Lipitor* are a $30 *billion* a year industry and they work very hard to push their myths in order to continue their sales. But I'm afraid that it just isn't as simple as the old "cholesterol gets too high and clogs your arteries and then you die" dogma. That's what they want you to believe, and that's the prevailing myth. Just about everybody believes it's true, but it's *not*. Studies show:

1) Cholesterol levels are a very poor predictor of heart attacks
2) 50% of people who have heart attacks have normal cholesterol levels
3) 50% of the people with elevated cholesterol have healthy hearts
4) dietary cholesterol (amount of cholesterol that you eat) makes very little difference in serum cholesterol levels.

Studies also indicate that lowering total cholesterol levels do not raise life expectations one bit. The world famous *Framingham Study* showed that those who developed heart disease and those who did not develop heart disease had virtually identical cholesterol levels.

The famous *Seven Countries Study* that gave birth to the "high cholesterol equals heart disease" myth was actually an extremely dishonest study. The study actually *involved 22 countries* (not seven!) and Ancel Keys, the man doing the study, **cherry picked** seven countries that best fit the hypothesis that he was working to support. In other words, he *lied* by using *biased* and *incomplete* data.

British doctor John Yudkin called him on his lie, and pointed out that there were other countries in the study that show identical levels of fats in their diets with totally different levels of heart disease, some of the 22 countries consumed lots of fat but had very little heart disease and vice versa; other countries consumed very little fat but had high rates of heart disease, which very quickly dispels the myth that cholesterol in diet has anything to do with heart disease. Consistency just didn't exist in that study when it came to correlations between fat intake, cholesterol levels and heart disease. As a matter of fact, the other famous study, *The Framingham Study*, showed that the *more* people *ate saturated fat, the lower* their serum cholesterol! You read that right. The people who ate the most fat had the lowest serum cholesterol levels! How's that for rocking the boat? Are you mad at me yet? I'm not making this stuff up, you can research it as much as you like. The data on those studies is out there. Go take a look!

The simple fact of the matter is that the level of serum cholesterol, your "total cholesterol" just doesn't make one damn bit of a difference. Your liver regulates cholesterol. If you eat less fat your liver will make more cholesterol. If you eat more fat your liver will make less cholesterol. Your body maintains the level of cholesterol that it needs! And yes, your body *needs* cholesterol! Nearly every cell in the human body contains cholesterol. Here's a quote from a fantastic book by one of my favorite doctors (take note that I didn't put quotes around the word "doctor" this time, because this man is a *real doctor* whom I have much respect for), Dr. Michael T. Murray, N.D. This is from his book *What the Drug Companies Won't Tell You, And What Your Doctor Doesn't Know*:

1. Cholesterol is used to form cell membranes; without it, cells lose their ability to function properly.

2. Cholesterol is a building block for Vitamin D and for many hormones, including cortisol, testosterone, progesterone, and estrogens.

3. Cholesterol is vital for proper neurological function, playing a role in memory and uptake of hormones in the brain.

Look at # 3 above; concerning brain function, although the brain only accounts for some 2% or 3% of total body weight, roughly *25% of total cholesterol is used by the brain.*

There is a study listed on *PubMed.gov* entitled *"Better memory functioning associated with higher total and low-density lipoprotein cholesterol levels in very elderly subjects without the apolipoprotein e4 allele"*. The title alone says it all. Their conclusion?

"...high cholesterol is associated with better memory function."

Full article is here: *http://www.ncbi.nlm.nih.gov/pubmed/18757771*

There's another article entitled *"Cholesterol-reducing Drugs May Lessen Brain Function, Says Researcher"* from

ScienceDaily.com that speaks for itself:

> "Yeon-Kyun Shin, a biophysics professor (at Iowa State University) in the department of biochemistry, biophysics and molecular biology, says the results of his study show that drugs that inhibit the liver from making cholesterol may also keep the brain from making cholesterol, which is vital to efficient brain function. 'If you deprive cholesterol from the brain, then you directly affect the machinery that triggers the release of neurotransmitters,' said Shin. 'Neurotransmitters affect the data-processing and memory functions. In other words -- how smart you are and how well you remember things.' Shin's findings will be published in this month's edition of the journal Proceedings of the National Academy of Sciences."

> **Full article is here**: *http://www.sciencedaily.com/releases/2009/02/090223221430.htm*

A book entitled *Lipitor Thief of Memory* by Duane Graveline, M.D. tells the story of a man who had very serious bouts with amnesia due to taking statin drugs and lowering his cholesterol too much. This is quoted from the book's *Amazon.com* page:

> "When Dr. Duane Graveline, former astronaut, aerospace medical research scientist, flight surgeon, and family doctor is given Lipitor to lower his cholesterol, he temporarily loses his short-term memory. Urged a year later to resume the drug at half dose, he lost both short-term and retrograde memory and was finally diagnosed in a hospital ER as having transient global amnesia (TGA). This is the 'scary, appealingly written' account of his search for answers that his medical community didn't have -- the how and why of his traumatic experience, and what needs to be done to prevent the devastating side effects to body and mind from the escalating use of the statin drugs."

As you can see, lowering your cholesterol too much can be very dangerous. Cholesterol is imperative to many bodily functions, *especially the brain*!

The powers that be do a damn good job of pounding it into people's heads that statin drugs "save lives because they lower cholesterol" but that's utter nonsense! Not even close. We've already seen what happens when you lower your cholesterol too much. Now let's take a look at some of the side effects of statin drugs.

A paper published in the *American Journal of Cardiovascular Drugs* entitled *"Statin Adverse Effects: A Review of the Literature and Evidence for a Mitochondrial Mechanism"* cites nearly **900 studies** on the adverse effects of statins! If that isn't enough to convince someone that these drugs are terribly, terribly toxic then what is? The *PubMed.gov* link is to the article is here: *http://www.ncbi.nlm.nih.gov/pmc/articles/PMC2849981*

Here is an *incomplete* list of the various side effects of these drugs:

- dizziness
- fainting
- fast or irregular heartbeat
- bladder pain
- bloody or cloudy urine
- blurred vision
- body aches or pain
- chills
- cough
- dark-colored urine
- difficult, burning, or painful urination
- difficulty with breathing
- difficulty with moving
- dry mouth
- ear congestion
- fever
- flushed, dry skin
- frequent urge to urinate
- fruit-like breath odor
- headache
- increased hunger
- increased thirst
- increased urination
- joint pain
- loss of consciousness
- lower back or side pain
- muscle cramps, spasms, or stiffness
- muscular pain, tenderness, wasting, or weakness
- nasal congestion
- nausea
- runny nose
- sneezing
- sore throat
- stomachache
- sweating
- swelling
- swollen joints
- troubled breathing
- unexplained weight loss
- unusual tiredness or weakness
- vomiting
- blistering, peeling, or loosening of the skin
- bloating
- burning, crawling, itching, numbness, prickling, "pins and needles", or tingling feelings
- constipation
- diarrhea
- difficulty with swallowing
- general tiredness and weakness
- indigestion
- large, hive-like swelling on the face, eyelids, lips, tongue, throat, hands, legs, feet, or
  sex - organs
- light-colored stools
- loss of appetite
- pains in the stomach, side, or abdomen, possibly radiating to the back
- pale skin
- puffiness or swelling of the eyelids or around the eyes, face, lips, or tongue
- red skin lesions, often with a purple center
- red, irritated eyes

- skin rash, hives, or itching
- sores, ulcers, or white spots in the mouth or on the lips
- tightness in the chest
- troubled breathing with exertion
- unusual bleeding or bruising
- upper right abdominal or stomach pain
- weakness in the arms, hands, legs, or feet
- yellow eyes or skin
- acid or sour stomach
- belching
- burning feeling in the chest or stomach
- dizziness or lightheadedness
- excess air or gas in the stomach or intestines
- feeling of constant movement of self or surroundings
- full feeling
- heartburn
- lack or loss of strength
- pain or tenderness around the eyes and cheekbones
- passing gas
- sensation of spinning
- skin rash, encrusted, scaly, and oozing
- stomach discomfort, upset, or pain
- tenderness in the stomach area
- trouble sleeping
- Incidence not known
- being forgetful
- depression
- discoloration of the skin
- hair loss or thinning of the hair
- inability to have or keep an erection
- loss in sexual ability, desire, drive, or performance

Whew! Now that's what I call a trade-off! All of that (plus more) for what benefit? Lowering cholesterol? Remember, "side effects" aren't side effects, they are *effects*. You might get an *effect* that you like, but you'll also get other *effects* that you don't like. Those negative *effects* happen because your body is telling you "Hey! Knock that shit off! Stop giving me this stuff!" If your body *wanted* toxic chemicals it wouldn't *protest*. And considering this long list of things that the body *protests* about with statin drugs, is there a good reason for taking these insane drugs? Obviously the human body doesn't think so!

And where's the evidence that lowering cholesterol prevents heart disease? Again; the famous *Framingham Study* clearly showed that those who developed heart disease and those who did *not* develop heart disease had *similar cholesterol levels. Also,* the 22 countries in the biased *Seven Country Study* showed that some of the countries with the *highest cholesterol levels* had the *least heart disease* and it's also a fact that 50% of the people who have heart attacks have cholesterol in the "normal" range. So please allow me to repeat myself one more time: *Where is the evidence that lowering cholesterol prevents heart disease? Where is the evidence that high cholesterol promotes it?* They have millions upon millions of people taking these very extremely dangerous drugs and they are raking in billions in profits annually, yet *there is no evidence that lowering cholesterol prevents heart disease!* Is this a crime against humanity? Well, go look at the list of side effects again and then answer that question for yourself. My answer is most definitely yes, it is a criminal act against humanity and an intentional fraud against innocent people who gullibly trust the establishment and "doctors".

So now you're probably sitting there scratching your head and thinking "Well Kenneth, if high cholesterol levels aren't responsible for heart disease, then what the hell is?" Your answer is as simple as one word: *Sugar*! Among other factors, but sugar is the main culprit, not cholesterol, thank you very much.

Aw yes. Sugar. This is the fun part for me because now I get to talk more about the diet that I feel so passionately about. I have said many things about low carb diets in this book, I've been praising them quite a bit in this book, I even went so far as to say this: *"There is no dietary lifestyle that is healthier than the low carbohydrate lifestyle."* Those are pretty strong claims, yes? Am I able to back up those claims with scientific evidence? Absolutely! I've already shown you the effect that the diet has upon diabetes and blood pressure, not to mention triglycerides. It basically cured my diabetes (as long as I stay on the diet), and yes, it has that effect in general with diabetes patients. A low carb diet also lowered my blood pressure significantly. I'm not making a "one size fits all" claim, or trying to say that there is only one diet for all people. But overall, a low car regimen is indeed healthier for the vast majority of all people unless they have special and/or rare health conditions that need to be addressed.

Over the years I've had many people question me on my diet and tell me "Kenny, you're going to die of a heart attack if you keep eating like that. You're eating nothing but saturated fat." And they're right, my diet is high in saturated fat. I eat lots of animal fats, I openly admit that. But if you were paying attention, I've already mentioned *twice* that in the famous *Framingham Study* the people who ate the most saturated fat had the *lowest* cholesterol levels! When I read that for the first time it didn't surprise me one bit, because I am no exception to that rule. Before I started the low carb lifestyle my total cholesterol was 266 and my triglycerides were a whopping 1414! After four months on the diet my total cholesterol had dropped down to 188 (within the "normal" range of mainstream "doctors") and my triglycerides had gone down to an amazing 233, an *84% reduction* in four months! **Repeat**: *Triglycerides took a nose dive from 1414 to 233 in four months on a diet high in saturated fat!* Are you mad at me yet?

Here's another one of my favorite doctors. He can explain this to you better than I can:

> "Logically, increased intake of fatty foods, such as greasy meats and butter, should increase blood triglycerides. This proved true, but only transiently and to a small degree. While increased intake of fats does does indeed deliver greater quantities of triglycerides into the liver and the bloodstream, it also shuts down the body's own production of triglycerides...the net effect is little or no change in triglyceride levels.
>
> Carbohydrates, on the other hand, contain virtually no triglycerides. But carbohydrates stimulate insulin, which in turn triggers fatty acid stimulus in the liver, a process that floods the bloodstream with triglycerides. Depending on genetic susceptibility, carbohydrates can send triglycerides into the hundreds or even thousands mg/dl range."
>
> - William Davis, M.D. (Author of *Wheat Belly*)

Something that I don't give a rat's ass about is the reduction of my total cholesterol from 266 to 188. As a matter of fact I'm a bit concerned that maybe it's too low, so I'm keeping an eye on that number.

Now let's talk about carbohydrates and sugar, which are one and the same as far as your body is concerned, and let's discuss the way in which carbohydrates and sugar affect your heart. First of all, carbs cause triglyceride production to go into overdrive, and when we're talking about triglycerides, we're talking about *heart disease*! Triglycerides are the biggest enemy of your heart. Period. Why is that? Well, because sugar and carbohydrates are the number one cause of high triglycerides. Sugar is sticky, it sticks to arterial walls, it causes inflammation and it oxidizes cholesterol. Cholesterol all by itself isn't a problem, but *oxidized* cholesterol certainly is, because oxidized cholesterol is sticky too. Sugar is sticky, triglycerides are sticky and oxidized cholesterol is sticky. When the arterial walls get damaged that creates inflammation and then "sticky things like to stick to it" which causes the dreaded plaque buildup that we all hear so much about. What causes damage to arterial walls? Well, sugar among other things. Yes, it went in a circle. And it always ends up at sugar. *Sugar causes inflammation and arterial damage, sugar causes high triglycerides and sugar oxidizes otherwise harmless cholesterol.* And remember, *carbohydrates are sugar (glucose)!*

Additionally, concerning so-called "good" (HDL) and "bad" (LDL) cholesterol, it isn't that simple:

There are two types of LDL ("bad") cholesterol; LDL-A, which are buoyant and fluffy molecules that do no harm whatsoever and LDL-B, which are small, hard, dense pellet like particles that promote atherosclerosis. So yes, *some* cholesterol is hazardous to your health. Total LDL levels are completely insignificant, it is only the type of LDL that makes a difference. You can have a high level of the buoyant and fluffy LDL-A and be just fine, or you can have an extremely low level of small, hard and dense pellet like LDL-B and definitely have something to be concerned about. And the same can be said for so-called "good" cholesterol (HDL). There is a "bad" kind and a "good" kind. Light and fluffy or hard and dense. Take your pick. The small, pellet like particles create tissue damage and oxidation as well as plaque buildup. Which brings us back to low carb diets; diets low in carbohydrates are shown to reduce the amount of the small, pellet like particles. Low carb diets in fact *create the larger fluffy kind* that are harmless!

And just think, I once had a "doctor" tell me that If I was going to be on a low carb diet long term, I could no longer be his patient. He refused to treat me any longer because I refused to stop the diet. He turned out to be dead *wrong* about low carb diets and his recommended diet (the standard low fat, high carb) has turned out to be a hazard to human health.

So far I've demonstrated that low carb diets:

1) Stabilize blood sugar in type 2 diabetics
2) Lower blood pressure
3) Lower triglycerides
4) Lower the small pellet like cholesterol particles
5) Create the harmless, big fluffy cholesterol particles instead
6) Increase energy
7) Reduce appetite
8) Improve health on all levels

I've also demonstrated that the diet most "doctors" want me to be on for diabetes, and the diet that is recommended by the *American Diabetes Association* (the standard low fat, high carb diet):

1) Increases blood glucose levels
2) Increases blood insulin levels
3) Raises blood pressure
4) Raises triglycerides
5) Creates more small, pellet like cholesterol particles
6) Promotes heart disease
7) Promotes obesity
8) Is *unquestionably* a hazard to human health!

I'm not making this stuff up. I have studies comparing low fat diets to low carb diets to prove it. Random controlled trials, the "gold standard" of science. Please see ___Appendix A___ in the back of the book. The data is clear, and I'll say it again; *there is no dietary lifestyle that is healthier than the low carbohydrate lifestyle*.

___What about vegan/vegetarian diets?___

I have encountered many vegans/vegetarians via the internet who like to arrogantly put themselves up on pedestals and scold people who eat meat, calling them "murderers" and such. I am always very quick to point out that those are religious/spiritual beliefs, nothing more. I tell them that if they don't want to eat animals because of their religious/spiritual beliefs then they are entitled to that belief and to that way of eating, but they have no right to judge others who do eat meat. I always point out that animals eating other animals is simply *nature* at work, it's called the *natural food chain*. If they get snippy with me I always pop back with a question similar to "What do you suggest, putting peace keeping troops in every jungle to stop the animals from eating each other?" Animals have been eating each other since the beginning of time, and just because vegans/vegetarians might not like it doesn't mean that it's going to change any time soon.

Vegans/vegetarians sometimes claim that the human body wasn't meant for meat, saying that humans are naturally herbivores, but that simply isn't true. Humans are omnivores, meaning that we eat both plants and meats, and that is backed by science. Even many vegetarians and vegans admit that fact. An article that was printed in the May/June 1991 edition of *Vegetarian*

Journal entitled *"Humans are Omnivores"* and written by a *vegetarian* named John McArdle, Ph.D. puts the biased and false claims that "humans are herbivores" to rest. The article, reprinted onto the website of the *Vegetarian Resource Group* is located here and the science is rock solid: https://www.vrg.org/nutshell/omni.htm

I also point out to vegans/vegetarians that their diets are not scientifically proven to be healthier than other diets, and that there are *no random controlled trials* or studies showing that their diets are healthier. To the contrary, vegan/vegetarian diets are often lacking in many important nutrients that can only be obtained from meats and proteins. Studies show that vegans/vegetarians are very commonly found to be deficient in Vitamin B12 in particular. Animal protein contains all of the essential amino acids in the right ratios, which are important to muscle mass and bone health, and of course vegans/vegetarians are lacking in those as well. Vegan/vegetarian diets are also low in creatine, carnosine and DHA, to name but a few. The list of nutrients that are lacking in vegan/vegetarian diets is, quite frankly, pretty long.

Vegans/vegetarians also typically consume **soy products** (tofu and others) regularly and swear by it as a healthy and stable source of protein, amino acids and other essential nutrients. The truth about soy is that it's not a complete protein, it lacks the amino acids methionine and cystine, 90% of it is genetically modified, and the list of health hazards of GMO foods is quite extensive, not to mention that manufacturers are legally permitted to mix GMO soy with just a little bit of truly organic soy and then label it as "organic", in other words, they're *legally permitted* to feed you GMO soy and call it "organic"! As for truly organic soy, just because it's "organic" doesn't mean that it's not a toxic poison, because, as a matter of fact, *it is*. Soy contains phytoestrogens, which are linked to increased infertility, various cancers and leukemia, as well as thyroid disease. They also lead to altered menstual cycles and in men, "man boobs", and they cause babies who are fed soy formulas to unnaturally develop faster as well as cause numerous health problems. In July of 1996, the *British Department of Health* issued a warning that the phytoestrogens found in soy baby formulas could cause health problems. Soy also contains trypsin inhibitors, which cause disorders of the pancreas and pancreatic cancer in rats. The hemagglutinin in soy causes red blood cells to clump together, potentially leading to blood clotting problems. Additionally, most "natural" food manufacturers are now using a toxic chemical called hexane to process their soy products. Hexane is the substance in glue that gets you high. It's also the part of gasoline that causes it to explode. And the last thing I'll mention about soy is that it contains phytic acid. Phytic acid blocks the uptake of essential minerals (calcium, magnesium, copper, iron and zinc). It basically deprives you of the nutrients that your body requires. It destroys bone health, blocking mineral absorption to the bones as well. Most scientists agree that diets high in phytic acid are largely responsible for mineral deficiencies in third world countries. Soy is not the "health food" that you think it is! Dr. William Wong states that *"Soy is poison, period!"* His article entitled *"Soy: The Poison Seed"* which lists numerous reasons for avoiding the poison that is soy, can be read at the following URL: *http://www.totalityofbeing.com/FramelessPages/Articles/SoyPoison.htm*

Vegans/vegetarians commonly quote a study called *The China Study* as so-called "proof" that their diets are healthier than other diets. *The China Study* was a twenty year long study conducted by *Cornell University's* Dr. Colin Campbell. He argued that the data suggests:

"People who ate the most animal-based foods got the most chronic disease...People who ate the most plant-based foods were the healthiest and tended to avoid chronic disease."

He made all of the data available in an 894-page book entitled *Diet, Lifestyle and Mortality in China* first printed in 1990.

A lady by the name of Denise Minger, a former vegan of over one full decade and author of the book *Death By Food Pyramid* analyzed the data and discovered that Dr. Campbell's conclusions were *incorrect* and were based upon incomplete (*cherry picked*) data. She said that she wasn't interested in trying to critique his conclusions until she discovered how untrue they are.

"My goal, with the China Study analysis and elsewhere, is to figure out the truth about nutrition and health without the interference of biases and dogma. I have no agenda to promote."

She discovered that Dr. Campbell conveniently ignored data that clearly shows correlations between wheat flour intake and coronary heart disease and weight gain. The graphs below are data compiled from Dr. Campbell's study that he never mentioned due to his bias in favor of vegan/vegetarian diets. The details of Ms. Minger's findings can be viewed on her website: *RawFoodSOS.com*

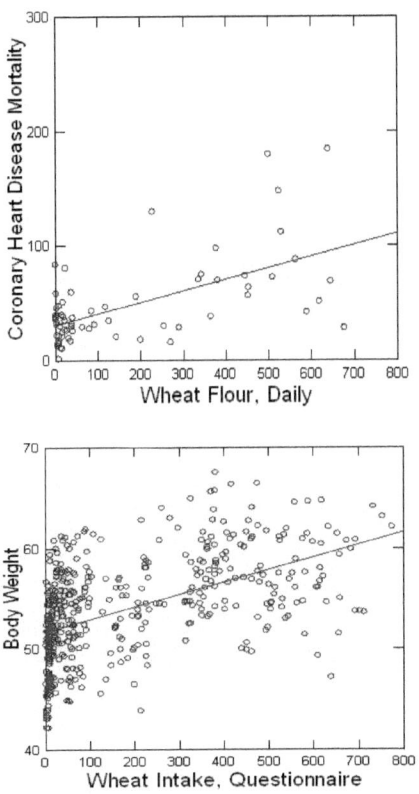

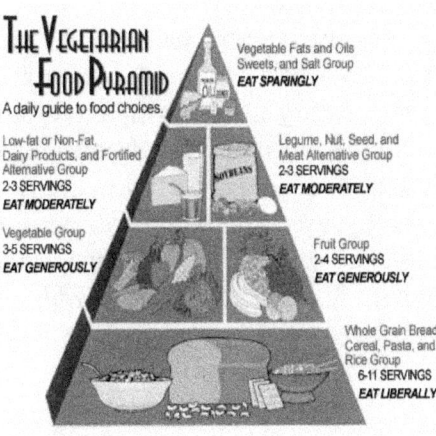

Vegan/vegetarian diets also typically embrace the "healthy whole grains" theory. Have a look above at the vegan/vegetarian food pyramid and see how chock-full it is with carbohydrates and wheat flour at the bottom, just like the USDA's pyramid. "6-11 servings daily, eat liberally". What have I been showing about carbohydrates and wheat consumption in this book so far? *Clearly this is not a healthy diet.*

Vegans/vegetarians typically demonize saturated fat in the diet as well, but I've already clearly demonstrated how important cholesterol is to every cell in the human body and especially brain function, and I've clearly shown that dietary cholesterol (amount of cholesterol you eat) has very little, if any impact at all, upon total serum cholesterol levels. The thing that I find amusing about their demonization of cholesterol is that their diet, because of all of the carbohydrates, actually *raises cholesterol*! Again, carbohydrates turn into pure glucose (sugar) after consumption, which raises triglycerides and cholesterol, blood glucose levels, blood insulin levels as well as blood pressure! I have clearly shown in this book that diets that are high in carbohydrates are *detrimental to human health on just about every level*. The science is clearly against vegan/vegetarian diets, it *most certainly is not a healthy way to eat.*
(Vegans/vegetarians can send all hate mail to: *kenny@loveevolvetranscend.com*)

Now; back to cholesterol. If you still aren't convinced that a high level of total serum cholesterol won't kill you, and if you still insist upon lowering your cholesterol, the first thing you need to know is this; don't lower it too much! We've already seen at the beginning of this section how the body depends on cholesterol and what can happen if it goes too low.

Secondly, you need to understand that drugs, especially seriously dangerous ones like *Lipitor* and other statins, are totally and completely unnecessary for lowering cholesterol. Here is a nice list of safe, natural and side effect free supplements that do just fine for achieving that goal. The following B-vitamins are extremely powerful for lowering both cholesterol and triglycerides. My personal preference is *Pantethine* because *Niacin* can sometimes cause harmless but very *unenjoyable* "flushing":

- Niacin (Vitamin B3)
- Pantethine (Vitamin B5)

Other supplements include:

- Borage Oil (GLA)
- Citrus bioflavanoids/tocotrienols (very popular in over the counter cholesterol supplements and very effective)
- Coconut Oil and/or "Medium Chain Fatty Acids"
- Cod Liver Oil (Omega-6 Fatty Acids)
- Fenugreek
- Fish Oil (Omega-3 Fatty Acids, EPA, DHA)
- Gugulipid
- Milk Thistle
- Psyllium Husks (high fiber intake)
- Vitamin A
- Vitamin C

There are more of course, but those are, by far, the most effective. **Pantethine** is really all you'd ever need, it's a miracle worker. If you want a replacement for statin drugs go with **Pantethine**. The citrus bioflavanoids/tocotrienols are very effective as well, they are the next best, but much more expensive. And in general, the more *fiber* in your diet, the *lower* your cholesterol will be.

Many people believe that taking *Red Yeast Rice* is good. It's true that it reduces cholesterol levels. But guess what? The main ingredient in statin drugs was isolated from *Red Yeast Rice* in US government funded labs in the 1970s. *Red Yeast Rice* is a statin drug, with all of the same side effects! Just say no to *Red Yeast Rice*! And even if you want to argue that point, the fact remains that it's not necessary to take *Red Yeast Rice* given all of the other options, so why bother with it?

"Doctors" rarely tell you this stuff, if ever, but let's not forget that they aren't really doctors, they are paid salespeople for drug companies masquerading as "medical professionals" that are interested in the well being of their clients. Ask yourself this question; if "doctors" were *truly* interested in the well being of their clients would they push deadly drugs first and foremost while they simultaneously blatantly ignore safe, natural and effective treatments? How exactly is the pushing of these dangerous cholesterol lowering drugs justified in the presence of things that work just as good, such as Pantethine, that are safe and side-effect free? My answer is that there is no justification, "doctors" and the medical establishment are a fraud and they are engaged in perpetuating a very deadly series of crimes against the majority of the common people in the interests of drug company profits and in their own financial interests as well in the form of kickbacks and payoffs from drug companies for being good salespeople. If they were truly "doctors" they'd live by the "first do no harm" ethic instead of living by the "first push drugs" rule that they engage in. You can accuse me of being too hard on them, but I'm really not. I'm pointing out something that is clearly true and I'm making a valid, unbiased observation. Yes, *some* of them mean well. *Some* of them really do care, but then they offer lousy care anyway because they're *ignorant*, which is just as bad, if not worse! If someone who went to college for seven years can't figure out that drugs cause their patients unnecessary harm then I'd say that there's something very, *very* wrong with this system of so-called "health care". The job of a doctor is to *provide the least harmful treatments possible*, because that's what *common sense* dictates! Why would any *real doctor* want to offer harmful and toxic treatments in the name of "health"? Isn't that just a glaringly obvious conflict of interest? A contradiction? Doesn't that go against all forms of sound logic? Poison for "health"? The only interest it serves is drug company profits, it certainly does *not* serve the best interests of the common people and it certainly does *not* promote health! Think about it!

Methicillin-resistant Staphylococcus (MRSA)

I was once employed by the mainstream medical establishment as a CNA (*Certified Nurse's Assistant*). I have since left that line of work due to my disgust with the medical system in general, and the fact that part of my job was passing out the drugs to the old folks. I always felt guilty doing that. I'd try to rationalize it in my mind telling myself things like "it's between them and their doctor, I'm just the middle man" and things like that, but ultimately I was never able to feel ok about it. I didn't like that part of the job at all. It wasn't uncommon for some of those old folks to be on six, seven or more drugs at the same time! I'd say the average number of drugs per resident in the homes I worked in was 4 or 5. Some of them had 10+ drugs that they took! And excuse the hell out of me, but *nobody* can tell me that drug pushing of that magnitude is necessary! They take advantage of old people and pile on the prescriptions because it makes them more money. "Doctors" get more kickbacks for more drugs prescribed, the drug companies make more money, and so on and so forth. Think of it on a national level. Think of all those nursing homes, adult family homes, etc. that are out there. That's a lot of drugs to be sold. And these old people really have no protections, their "doctors" will prescribe them with drugs and there's never an opportunity for these folks to refuse or say no. In some cases, sure, but most of them are totally leaving everything up to their "doctor" and many of them are simply too out of it to pay any attention. The nursing homes of the country are very much abusing our old folks by drugging them far, *far* beyond what is required, but nobody seems to notice and nobody seems to care. It's business as usual. And sadly, if I were to mention this to the people who work in these homes, the nurses, the CNA's, etc., the vast majority would argue and deny. *Argue and deny.* Why? Because they're robots serving the system, non-thinking obedient workers doing as they're told and then going home to watch football and drink beer with their families. "Don't forget your medicine dear. Did you take your Prozac today?" They're all mindlessly serving the system with no conscience and no remorse, basically. People like me *with a conscience* are obviously quite rare. Additionally, many of the nurses and CNA's I worked with were cold and hardened. They'd been doing it for years and as a result they'd become totally insensitive and cold. Some of them were downright **mean** to the old people. And that wasn't an uncommon thing, *many of them were that way*, and I found it disgusting and repulsive. It broke my heart. I was there to give the old folks some loving care, and then I saw that happening. If you can avoid sending your loved ones to nursing homes they'll be much better off. I do not recommend nursing homes. If you're hard pressed to find a place for someone, smaller adult family homes, depending upon who runs it, would be a better option. I've worked in those places too, and you get much more personalized and friendlier care because of the smaller staff and the fact that there are far less residents to care for, the maximum capacity generally being 6 residents. Larger nursing homes should be avoided like the plague. Trust me, stay away from those if you want decent care for your loved one!

I didn't like that line of work but it did serve as a learning experience for me. Not only did I gain inside knowledge into the system and how things work, I was forced to learn how to deal with the terrible consequence of being exposed to patients with antibiotic resistant staph infections because I was somehow given a *MRSA* infection during the course of my work by one of the residents. As quoted from *WebMD.com*:

"What Is MRSA?

Methicillin-resistant Staphylococcus aureus (MRSA) is a bacterium that causes infections in different parts of the body. It's tougher to treat than most strains of staphylococcus aureus -- or staph -- because it's resistant to some commonly used antibiotics.

The symptoms of MRSA depend on where you're infected. Most often, it causes mild infections on the skin, like sores or boils. But it can also cause more serious skin infections or infect surgical wounds, the bloodstream, the lungs, or the urinary tract.

Though most MRSA infections aren't serious, some can be life-threatening. Many public health experts are alarmed by the spread of tough strains of MRSA. Because it's hard to treat, MRSA is sometimes called a 'super bug.'"

Full article is here: *http://www.webmd.com/skin-problems-and-treatments/understanding-mrsa-methicillin-resistant-staphylococcus-aureus*

MRSA was created by the over-use and over-prescribing of antibiotics. "Doctors" routinely pass out antibiotics quickly and without much thought at all, even when it's not an appropriate treatment. The fact of the matter is that antibiotics do not help one bit when you're dealing with a virus such as a cold, cough or flu. The following is quoted straight from the FDA's website:

"Using them for viruses will not make you feel better or get back to work faster. Antibiotics are strong medicines. Keep them that way. Prevent antibiotic resistance. Antibiotics don't fight viruses – they fight bacteria. Using antibiotics for viruses can put you at risk of getting a bacterial infection that is resistant to antibiotic treatment. Talk to your doctor or other healthcare provider about antibiotics, visit www.cdc.gov/getsmart, or call 800-CDC-INFO (800-232-4636) to learn more."

Full article is here: http://www.fda.gov/Drugs/ResourcesForYou/ucm078494.htm

Despite the warnings even from the FDA in this case, "doctors" still pass out antibiotics like candy, for every reason under the sun, which has led to huge outbreaks of antibiotic resistant strains of staphylococcus aureus (staph infections). The CDC (*Centers for Disease Control and Prevention*) reported on September 18, 2003 that the number of unnecessary antibiotics prescribed annually for viral infections was in the **tens of millions**.

My MRSA experience started one morning when I got out of bed, went to the shower and noticed huge boils with kind of sharp prickly points all over my belly. When I say huge I mean maybe half the size of a golf ball. They were kind of like chickenpox, but about ten times larger, and they were all over my belly area, I'd guess about 20 to 30 of them. I immediately called in sick for work and then went straight to the emergency room. They did some tests, confirmed MRSA, gave me antibiotics and sent me on my way. Within a few days I was ok again, no more boils, and ignorantly believing that I was done dealing with MRSA. It didn't work out that way. Within six weeks I had boils popping up on my head, this time not so big and not so many of them, but clearly there was a problem. I didn't know what else to do, so I went to ER again. As expected, all they did was give me another round of antibiotics and send me on my way. The boils went away again, and then came back *again* about four to six weeks later. Once again, I knew not what to do! I was ignorant at this point on how to deal with MRSA and had no idea how hard it would be to get rid of.

During the course of a year or so, I was intermittently dealing with these boils and sores popping up all over my body. At one point I had a baseball sized abscess on the left cheek of my ass and had to go to ER to have it drained. I had another abscess on my forearm that I drained myself. I knew what it was and how to deal with it because of the one that I had on my ass. It was getting real tiring dealing with all of these boils and sores, and I was worried that maybe something could happen to me *internally* as well. Thinking back on this, I do believe that I'm lucky to be alive because I very easily could have had MRSA infections, boils, etc on *internal organs*. That's how bad it was. Those sores were popping up everywhere, and I feel lucky to be alive, no thanks to "doctors" because they did **nothing** to help me at all!

I knew that "doctors" would only give me more antibiotics and send me packing again, so in my desperation I started scouring the internet looking for solutions. After a few days of searching high and low for answers to my problem, looking at forums and websites all over the internet, I finally managed to find my solution.

Before I share with you how I kicked MRSA's ass, I want to share something with you about antibiotics. This is quoted from an article entitled *"Antibiotics Put 142,000 Into Emergency Rooms Each Year: U.S. Centers for Disease Control Waits 60 Years to Study the Problem"*:

"OMNS, October 13, 2008) The US Centers for Disease Control (CDC) has just released 'the first report ever done on adverse reactions to antibiotics in the United States' on 13 Aug, 2008. This is 'the first report ever'? How is that possible? Antibiotics have been widely used since the 1940s. It is astounding that it has taken CDC so long to seriously study the side effects of these drugs. It is now apparent that there have been decades of an undeserved presumption of safety.

Antibiotics can put you in the emergency room. Common antibiotics, the ones most frequently prescribed and regarded as safest, cause nearly half of emergencies due to antibiotics. And, incredibly enough, people in the prime of life - not babies - are especially at risk. The study authors reported that 'Persons aged 15-44 years accounted for an estimated 41.2 percent of emergency department visits. Infants accounted for only an estimated 6.3 percent of ED visits.' They also found that nearly 80% of antibiotic-caused 'adverse events' were allergic reactions. Overdoses and mistakes, by patients and by physicians, make up the rest.

Allergic reactions to antibiotics may be very serious, including life-threatening anaphylactic shock. Searching the US National Library of Medicine's 'Medline' database for 'antibiotic allergic reaction' will bring up over 9,700 mentions in scientific papers. A search for 'antibiotic anaphylactic shock' brings up over 1,100. Many papers on this severe danger were actually published before 1960. Given this amount of accumulated information, one might wonder why CDC took so long to seriously study the problem.

Overuse of antibiotics leads to antibiotic resistance. At its website, CDC currently states that antibiotic resistance 'can cause significant danger and suffering for people who have common infections that once were easily treatable with antibiotics. . .Some resistant infections can cause death.'

In the USA alone, 'over 3 million pounds of antibiotics are used every year on humans . . .enough to give every man, woman and child 10 teaspoons of pure antibiotics per year,' write Null, Dean, Feldman, and Rasio. 'Almost half of patients with upper respiratory tract infections in the U.S. still receive antibiotics from their doctor' even though 'the CDC warns that 90% of upper respiratory infections, including children's ear infections, are viral, and antibiotics don't treat viral infection. More than 40% of about 50 million prescriptions for antibiotics each year in physicians' offices were inappropriate.'"

Full article is here: *http://orthomolecular.org/resources/omns/v04n14.shtml*

Clearly antibiotics are not all they are claimed to be. *Clearly* they are dangerous. *Clearly* they are toxic. *Clearly* they need to be avoided unless absolutely necessary. I'm not opposed to using antibiotics in emergency situations, they can and do save lives, but the vast majority of the time antibiotics are totally unnecessary and at the end of this section I will give you many examples of safe, natural and side effect free herbs and supplements with antibiotic properties that can replace these dangerous drugs.

An interesting tidbit of information concerning antibiotics is that they cause yeast infections. How, you ask? Well, your stomach and intestines contain bacteria, "good" bacteria (beneficial flora) and "bad" bacteria, one of those being Candida (yeast, fungus). When you take antibiotics it kills *all* bacteria, including the good stuff. When the good bacteria gets too low there is no longer protection against the bad bacteria, leaving Candida with a free pass to do whatever it wants. If you do take antibiotics for whatever reason, always make sure that you're also taking a *probiotic* for support. Probiotics give your stomach and intestines the good bacteria that it needs, restoring balance to the system. As I said before, antibiotics kill *all* bacteria indiscriminately, but the *natural* antibiotic that I used to kick MRSA's ass (and the antibiotic herbs that I will list off) *only kill the bad bacteria* leaving the good bacteria intact!

Here is the information that you need to know regarding a natural alternative to antibiotic drugs, especially if you have staph infections like MRSA!

As quoted from *ColloidalSilverCuresMRSA.com*:

"Criminalizing the Cure for MRSA!

You see, instead of alerting the public to the cure for MRSA, the health authorities have instead waged a long, intractable warfare against it for the past 30 years. Indeed, the cure for MRSA was originally discovered by Dr. Robert O. Becker, M.D. during his groundbreaking research into 'incurable' infections at Syracuse Medical University, way back in the 1970's!

Dr. Becker used the simple cure he had discovered to heal every 'incurable' infection they brought to him, without fail. He even published the results of his research in peer-reviewed medical journals, knowing that what he had discovered would, quite literally, change the world.

He had been attempting to demonstrate his theory that small micro-currents of electricity could be used to make stubborn infected bone fractures heal completely. And during the course of his experiments, he began using silver electrodes in order to take advantage of silver's well-known propensity to conduct electricity. But what he discovered in the process took him completely by surprise.

You see, not only did the micro-currents of electricity trigger the bone fractures to heal just as he had expected, but the tiny, electrically generated silver particles that were driven into the bone and surrounding tissue from the silver electrodes healed ALL nearby infections. Even rare and potentially deadly infections such as osteomyelitis were rapidly healed!

Dr. Becker later concluded:

'What we have done was rediscover the fact that silver kills bacteria, a fact which had actually been known for centuries ...All of the organisms we tested were sensitive to the electrically generated silver ion, including some that were resistant to all known antibiotics...In no case were any undesirable side effects of the silver treatment apparent.'

Yes, indeed. Dr. Becker had re-discovered a fact that medical researchers of old had once known, but that had become lost to medicine ever since the age of prescription antibiotic drugs had been ushered in by the global pharmaceutical conglomerates during the 1930's and 40's. He had re-discovered the fact that silver – one of the world's oldest and most powerful natural antibiotic substances – could kill just about any pathogen exposed to it. Even the most virulent of pathogens succumb to it with ease!

But instead of accolades, he received anonymity. His research was shunned. And his funding was cut off. To alert the world to his findings, he published two books in the 1980's and early 1990's – The Body Electric and Cross Currents – both of which went on to become NY Times and LA Times bestsellers.

But since that time, the medical authorities have clamped down on information about the cure for MRSA. In fact, they have actually passed laws restricting information about it, even to the point of making it a criminal offense to tell the public about the cure for these deadly super-pathogens. It's astonishing. Yet it's absolutely true!"

Full article is here: *http://www.colloidalsilvercuresmrsa.com/mrsa_cure.htm*

Once again, the drug pushing profit makers don't want to lose business, and so they suppress valuable, life saving information in order to preserve their profit margins.

When I discovered this information via their website, the first thing that I did was run as fast as I could to a health food store. I found some colloidal silver and purchased it immediately. I was infected at the time, so I started out on pretty high doses. I took about a shot glass (1 ½ oz each) full of 10 ppm (parts per million) colloidal silver three times daily, and as expected the boils went away. Not only did the boils go away, they went away almost immediately, much faster than they had previously with the antibiotics from ER.

I was very happy with my results but the health food store

silver was too expensive. It didn't take me long to discover that I could easily make the stuff for only pennies per gallon. I started producing my own with distilled water, silver wire and a 9-volt battery. I have now been taking about two tablespoons per day of colloidal silver for nearly five years and with the exception of a couple of bouts with upper respiratory infections due to breathing in too much cold air during the winter, I have not been sick one day. Colloidal silver is a natural antibiotic, but unlike prescription antibiotics, colloidal silver will not only leave the good bacteria alone, it will kill viruses too! See the following website: *ColloidalSilverKillsViruses.com*

Before I started taking colloidal silver every day I would get sick at least once a year with strep throat, flu and things like that. Not any more! Not for five years now!

I would like to share with you some excerpts from my first book *LOVE - EVOLVE - TRANSCEND: Building a Spiritual Culture on the Planet Earth.* This is from the chapter entitled *"Naturopathic and Electric Medicine: The Wave of the Future"*:

"Electricity is the basis for much of what is going to be the new paradigm in medicine when the new spiritual culture upon the planet Earth emerges and the lies of the current mainstream 'medicine' are exposed. Interestingly, there is no profit to be made from any of these therapies, which is not only why they aren't practiced today, it's also why these discoveries are being suppressed. Unlike today's vaccines and antibiotics which are full of poisonous, deadly toxins and heavy metals such as mercury, formaldehyde, aluminum, anti-freeze, etc. and called 'medicine' by the medical establishment, electricity effectively kills all harmful, disease causing bacteria, as does oxygen. Ionic (electrically charged) silver is known to kill all disease causing bacteria inside of six minutes in every test that has ever been conducted in laboratories, and it is totally nontoxic:

'Placing colloidal particles of silver into a beaker of water that contains bacteria will kill the bacteria. Placing these colloidal silver particles in a nearby gas discharge tube, and focusing the electromagnetic emissions from such an operating tube onto the beaker, will also kill the bacteria. Via this simple example we see that it is the specific information pattern inherent in the silver atom and not the physical contact that is killing the bacteria.' - William A. Tiller, Stanford University, Professor Emeritus of Materials Science, author of Science and Human Transformation: Subtle Energies, Intentionality and Consciousness.

As we can see from the above paragraph, physical contact with the silver is not necessary in order to kill bacteria, it is the electromagnetic emission from the silver that kills the bacteria, not the silver itself. It is the electrical nature of the silver that is causing the harmful bacteria to be eliminated.

Colloidal Silver: Home-made, pennies-per-gallon colloidal silver acts as a 'second immune system.' It has been shown in numerous studies to be the only substance known to eliminate hundreds of viruses, bacteria, fungus, etc., more than any modern antibiotic or 'miracle drug' yet developed by the pharmaceutical companies. It greatly assists in eliminating pathogens and guards against opportunistic infections. It can be used anywhere in or on the body.

Kenneth C. Dyer, Jr.

Patents:

1973: Patent # 7135195: 'Treatment of Humans With Colloidal Silver Composition'

Colloidal silver generators are as low as $49.00 on the internet, just go to Google and search.

Colloidal Silver: The Universal Antibiotic

(This was compiled from Bob Beck's free paper 'Take Back Your Power' which is available on the internet. I added in some things as well.)

No known disease-causing organism can live in the presence of even minute traces of colloidal silver, and there are zero negative side effects! Do you have an antibiotic in your home emergency preparedness kit? How about a way to purify contaminated water? You can make colloidal silver at home for free quickly, easily and legally. And when you stop to consider the fact that vaccines and antibiotics are pumped full of toxic poisons such as mercury (the most poisonous substance known to humankind!), aluminum, formaldehyde, antifreeze, and numerous other ludicrous, inexcusable ingredients, doesn't it make you wonder why they've been keeping colloidal silver a secret while they make their millions of dollars in profits selling you their toxic waste, I mean 'medicine'? Imagine, just for a second, if everyone knew about the benefits of colloidal silver. What do you think that would do to the profits of these industries? And don't forget that many of the people in government have financial ties to the very companies that produce and sell the vaccines and antibiotics, as well as the medical establishment. The people in power are the people hiding the cures. The system that is in place is about making money and corporate profits, not about helping people. They rely upon people being sick to make their money. Every time someone is cured they lose a customer. Sad but true, the system that is in place today must be abolished.

What is Colloidal Silver?

A colloid refers to a substance that consists of ultra-fine particles that do not dissolve, but remain suspended in a medium of different matter. These ultra-fine particles are larger than most molecules but so small they cannot be seen by the naked eye. Colloidal silver is not a chemical compound containing silver, but a pure metallic silver of sub-microscopic clusters of just a few atoms, held in suspension, in pure water, by the tiny electric charge on each atom. In short, colloidal silver is simply teeny, tiny particles of silver suspended in purified water, nothing else.

Colloidal silver was in common use until 1938. Many people remember their grandparents putting silver dollars in milk to prolong its freshness at room temperature. At the turn of the century, scientists had discovered that the body's most important fluids are colloidal in nature: suspended ultra-fine particles. Blood, for example, carries nutrition and oxygen to the body cells. This led to studies with colloidal silver. Prior to 1938, colloidal silver was used by physicians as a mainstream antibiotic treatment and was considered quite 'high-tech.' Production methods, however, were costly. The pharmaceutical industry moved in, causing colloidal research to be set aside in favor of financially lucrative drugs. The FDA classifies colloidal silver as a pre-1938 drug. A letter from the FDA dated 9/13/91 states: 'These products may continue to be marketed as long as they are advertised and labeled for the same use as in 1938 and as long as they are manufactured in the original manner.'

Most Important Qualities:

Colloidal Silver is a powerful, natural antibiotic, used for thousands of years, with no known side effects. This was used by medical doctors before the invention of mainstream conventional antibiotics which are far less effective. Colloidal Silver is a catalyst, disabling the particular enzyme that all one-celled bacteria, fungus and virus, use for their oxygen metabolism. It is of no harm to human enzymes or any part of the human body chemistry. It can kill all disease-causing organisms, in six minutes or less, upon contact, no matter how they mutate. Resistant strains, such as MRSA, fail to develop, and the body doesn't develop a tolerance. The best possible treatment for MRSA, which is being silenced by the mainstream press, the pharmaceutical industry, and the medical community is colloidal silver! *www.colloidalsilvercuresmrsa.com*. Colloidal Silver is both a remedy and a prevention of infections of all kinds. Having sufficient Colloidal Silver in your body is to have a superior, second immune system. Non-toxic, no known side effects, is made entirely from the pure mineral element, silver · Contains no chemicals or proteins · Useful against over 650 disease-causing organisms (i.e. germs, fungi & some viruses) · Helps strengthen the body's natural defenses (when taken daily), is highly germicidal · Helps growth stimulation of injured tissues, is a remedy for infections · May be used internally or applied topically. The following is a partial list of the more than 650 diseases that Colloidal Silver has been known to have been used successfully against: abrasion • leukemia • acne • lupus • acne • AIDS • lyme disease • allergies • malaria • appendicitis • meningitis • arthritis • mosquito bites • athlete's foot • bladder inflammation • parasitic infections (viral & fungal) • blood parasites • pneumonia • blood poisoning • boils • prostate • bubonic plague • burns •psoriasis • cancer • chronic fatigue • scarlet fever • colds/flu • shingles • dermatitis • skin cancer • diabetes • sores • dysentery • staph infections • eczema • syphilis • thyroid • gastritis • tonsillitis • gonorrhea • hay fever • herpes • tuberculosis • indigestion • virus (all forms) • infections • warts • inflammations • whooping-cough • itchy skin • yeast infection + more!

An excellent website to read about the modern scientific studies of colloidal silver is here: *www.thesilveredge.com/sources.shtml*.

Based on laboratory tests with colloidal silver, destructive bacteria, virus, and fungus organisms are killed within minutes of contact. Larry C. Ford, M.D, of the Department of Obstetrics and Gynecology, UCLA School of Medicine, Center For The Health Sciences reported in a letter dated November 1, 1988, 'I tested the silver solutions using standard antimicrobial tests for disinfectants. The silver solutions were antibacterial for concentrations of 10 organisms per ml. of Streptococcus Pyogenes, Staphylococcus Aurcus, Neisseria Gonorrhea, Gardnerella Vaginalis, Salmonella Typhi, and other enteric pathogens, and fungicidal for Candida Albicans, Candida Globata, and M. Furfur.' Jim Powell reported in a Science Digest article March, 1978, titled, 'Our Mightiest Germ Fighter,' 'Thanks to eye-opening research, silver is emerging as a wonder of modern medicine. An antibiotic kills perhaps a half-dozen different disease organisms, but silver kills some 650. Resistant strains fail to develop, moreover, silver is virtually non-toxic.' Dr. Harry Margraf of St. Louis concluded 'Silver is the best all around germ-fighter we have.' UCLA Medical Center has reported that 'colloidal silver killed every virus that was tested in the lab.' Dr. Henry Crooks, speaking about colloidal silver, states: 'I know of no microbe that is not killed in laboratory experiments in six minutes.' Dr. Harry Margraf of St. Louis states: 'Colloidal silver is the best all-around germ fighter we have.' Colloidal Silver has been found to be both a remedy and prevention for all colds, all flu, all infections and all fermentation due to any bacteria, fungus or virus, especially staph and strep, which are found present in many disease conditions.

How To Use It

Applications include oral, topical, by injection, as a nasal, ear, or eye drop, or as a spray for other sensitive tissues. Since it kills all disease causing bacteria, fungi, and virus within six minutes of contact but leaves unharmed the 'friendly' bacteria, many people take it internally every day as a boost for their immune system. It does not sting, burn, or otherwise hurt even the most sensitive areas, even a baby's eyes. It can be used on warts, open sores, or a rinse for acne, eczema, and other skin irritations. It can be used vaginally, anally, or even atomized and inhaled.

Make It At Home For Free

The FDA has no jurisdiction over a pure mineral element therefore colloidal silver can be purchased over the counter at many health food stores and can also be legally made by you for free in the privacy of your own home. It is very quick and easy.

The Hype

The same people who don't want you to know about this because it would affect their profits are putting out a propaganda campaign against it. When they encounter people who know about it and use it they are quick to put out misinformation claiming that colloidal silver causes a condition known as 'argyria' which turns the skin grey and/or blue. But the truth is that: 'Out of the estimated 10 million regular users of colloidal silver throughout North America today, there have been fewer than 120 documented cases of argyria in the past 50 years. Most of these were caused by the ingestion of liquid chemical compounds of silver, rather than properly made, electrically generated colloidal silver.' - *'The Ultimate Colloidal Silver Manual'* published by Life & Health Research Group, LLC; 1-888-846-9029; *www.lifeandhealthresearchgroup.com*

In other words, made properly, with nothing but distilled water and pure silver wire, the chances of getting argyria from colloidal silver are less than the chance of being struck by lightning. So don't believe the hype!"

Long after I nipped MRSA in the bud with colloidal silver I learned of other natural MRSA fighters (but I still firmly believe that colloidal silver is the most effective by a long shot). The vast majority of these also function as *antivirals*:

- Garlic (powerful antibiotic, but **remember that it is toxic**)
- Olive Leaf Extract (used in Hungarian hospitals to treat MRSA)
- Oregano Oil (powerful antibiotic)
- Organic Honey (Manuka Honey in particular)
- Pascalite (bentonite clay found only in mountains of Wyoming)
- Tea Tree Oil (powerful antibacterial)
- Turmeric (powerful antibacterial)

There are, of course, numerous herbs that act as antibiotics. Most of these are also *antivirals*:

- Achornea
- Andrographis
- Artemisia
- Ashwaganda
- Astragalus
- Barberry
- Bidens
- Boneset
- Cordyceps
- Cryptolepis
- Echinacea
- Elderberry
- Eleuthero
- Ginger
- Goldenseal Root
- Juniper
- Licorice
- Red Root
- Reishi
- Rhodiola
- Sida

There are more, but these are the most powerful by a long shot. As you can see, there are many natural ways to combat the "incurable" MRSA. If you ever pick up a MRSA infection you'll only do more damage to yourself if you use antibiotics, and then the MRSA will just come right back a month or two later, so do yourself a favor, **<u>use colloidal silver and do it right the first time</u>**!

The great MRSA cover-up is just another in a long list of criminal, murderous acts perpetuated by mainstream medicine and Big Pharma. I'm not through yet. The crimes get much worse.

Depression

I battled with depression quite a bit during my late 20s and early 30s. At one point I spent about five years wishing I was dead, but I wasn't miserable enough to actually do anything about it. I was thinking "if only someone would do me a favor and shoot me in the back of the head, that would be great".

I never sought treatment for depression, so I have no stories to tell about my experiences with "doctors" on this issue, and for the most part I've been happy since I was introduced to Reiki, which is a form of energy healing that you can read about in *Appendix B*.

I have been involved in Reiki healing since 1997 and it has made a tremendous difference in my life, as a matter of fact I give it credit for quite literally saving my life. My book *LOVE - EVOLVE - TRANSCEND: Building a Spiritual Culture on the Planet Earth* details my story on how I was introduced to Reiki and how it came to matter so much to me. Reiki healing was *definitely* the "cure" for my depression.

Additionally, when I switched from synthetic T4-only thyroid medication to NDT (natural desiccated thyroid) I did notice an elevation in my moods as well, because one symptom of hypothyroidism is depression, and my thyroid was out of whack. Once I corrected the thyroid levels, I experienced happier moods.

Knowing what I now know about so-called "antidepressant" drugs makes me very glad that I never sought treatment or took any of those drugs. Antidepressant drugs are associated with suicidal thoughts and batshit crazy behavior. They do more damage to people than anything else. They have severe side effects, which I will list off soon, and even the FDA issued the following which can be seen on their website:

"Antidepressant Use in Children, Adolescents, and Adults

[5/2/2007] The U.S. Food and Drug Administration (FDA) today proposed that makers of all antidepressant medications update the existing black box warning on their products' labeling to include warnings about increased risks of suicidal thinking and behavior, known as suicidality, in young adults ages 18 to 24 during initial treatment (generally the first one to two months).

List of Antidepressant Drugs with Medication Guides

Anafranil (clomipramine)
Asendin (amoxapine)

Aventyl (nortriptyline)
Celexa (citalopram hydrobromide)
Cymbalta (duloxetine)
Desyrel (trazodone HCl)
Elavil (amitriptyline)
Effexor (venlafaxine HCl)
Emsam (selegiline)
Etrafon (perphenazine/amitriptyline)
fluvoxamine maleate
Lexapro (escitalopram oxalate)
Limbitrol (chlordiazepoxide/amitriptyline)
Ludiomil (maprotiline)
Marplan (isocarboxazid)
Nardil (phenelzine sulfate)
nefazodone HCl
Norpramin (desipramine HCl)
Pamelor (nortriptyline)
Parnate (tranylcypromine sulfate)
Paxil (paroxetine HCl)
Pexeva (paroxetine mesylate)
Prozac (fluoxetine HCl)
Remeron (mirtazapine)
Sarafem (fluoxetine HCl)
Seroquel (quetiapine)
Sinequan (doxepin)
Surmontil (trimipramine)
Symbyax (olanzapine/fluoxetine)
Tofranil (imipramine)
Tofranil-PM (imipramine pamoate)
Triavil (perphenazine/amitriptyline)
Vivactil (protriptyline)
Wellbutrin (bupropion HCl)
Zoloft (sertraline HCl)
Zyban (bupropion Hcl)"

Full article is here: _http://www.fda.gov/Drugs/_
DrugSafety/InformationbyDrugClass/ucm096273.htm

Yes, they *"cause suicidal thoughts"* and they cause people to quite literally go off the deep end as well! Allow me to illustrate my point with quotes from _NaturalNews.com_'s website, in a story entitled *"Every Mass Shooter in the Last 20 Years Has One Thing In Common, And It's Not Guns"*:

"The overwhelming evidence points to the single largest common factor in all of these incidents...the fact that all of the perpetrators were either actively taking powerful psychotropic drugs or had been at some point in the immediate past before they committed their crimes.

Multiple credible scientific studies going back more then a decade, as well as internal documents from certain pharmaceutical companies that suppressed the information show that SSRI drugs (Selective Serotonin Re-Uptake Inhibitors) have well known, but unreported side effects, including but not limited to suicide and other violent behavior. One need only Google relevant key words or phrases to see for themselves. www.ssristories.com is one popular site that has documented over 4500 "Mainstream Media" reported cases from around the World of aberrant or violent behavior by those taking these powerful drugs.

The following (is a) list of mass shooting perpetrators and the drugs they were taking or had been taking shortly before their horrific actions. I leave it to the individual readers to make up their own minds if...the list of mass shooters...link to psychotropic drugs:

• Eric Harris age 17 (first on Zoloft then Luvox) and Dylan Klebold aged 18 (Columbine school shooting in Littleton, Colorado), killed 12 students and 1 teacher, and wounded 23 others, before killing themselves. Klebold's medical records have never been made available to the public.

• Jeff Weise, age 16, had been prescribed 60 mg/day of Prozac (three times the average starting dose for adults!) when he shot his grandfather, his grandfather's girlfriend and many fellow students at Red Lake, Minnesota. He then shot himself. 10 dead, 12 wounded.

• Cory Baadsgaard, age 16, Wahluke (Washington state) High School, was on Paxil (which caused him to have hallucinations) when he took a rifle to his high school and held 23 classmates hostage. He has no memory of the event.

• Chris Fetters, age 13, killed his favorite aunt while taking Prozac.

• Christopher Pittman, age 12, murdered both his grandparents while taking Zoloft.

• Mathew Miller, age 13, hung himself in his bedroom closet after taking Zoloft for 6 days.

• Kip Kinkel, age 15, (on Prozac and Ritalin) shot his parents while they slept then went to school and opened fire killing 2 classmates and injuring 22 shortly after beginning Prozac treatment.

• Luke Woodham, age 16 (Prozac) killed his mother and then killed two students, wounding six others.

• A boy in Pocatello, ID (Zoloft) in 1998 had a Zoloft-induced seizure that caused an armed stand off at his school.

• Michael Carneal (Ritalin), age 14, opened fire on students at a high school prayer meeting in West Paducah, Kentucky. Three teenagers were killed, five others were wounded..

• A young man in Huntsville, Alabama (Ritalin) went psychotic chopping up his parents with an ax and also killing one sibling and almost murdering another.

• Andrew Golden, age 11, (Ritalin) and Mitchell Johnson, aged 14, (Ritalin) shot 15 people, killing four students, one teacher, and wounding 10 others.

• TJ Solomon, age 15, (Ritalin) high school student in Conyers, Georgia opened fire on and wounded six of his class mates.

• Rod Mathews, age 14, (Ritalin) beat a classmate to death with a bat.

• James Wilson, age 19, (various psychiatric drugs) from Breenwood, South Carolina, took a .22 caliber revolver into an elementary school killing two young girls, and wounding seven other children and two teachers.

• Elizabeth Bush, age 13, (Paxil) was responsible for a school shooting in Pennsylvania

• Jason Hoffman (Effexor and Celexa) – school shooting in El Cajon, California

• Jarred Viktor, age 15, (Paxil), after five days on Paxil he stabbed his grandmother 61 times.

Drugging for "Health": Why the Paradigm Must Change

• Chris Shanahan, age 15 (Paxil) in Rigby, ID who out of the blue killed a woman.

• Jeff Franklin (Prozac and Ritalin), Huntsville, AL, killed his parents as they came home from work using a sledge hammer, hatchet, butcher knife and mechanic's file, then attacked his younger brothers and sister.

• Neal Furrow (Prozac) in LA Jewish school shooting reported to have been court-ordered to be on Prozac along with several other medications.

• Kevin Rider, age 14, was withdrawing from Prozac when he died from a gunshot wound to his head. Initially it was ruled a suicide, but two years later, the investigation into his death was opened as a possible homicide. The prime suspect, also age 14, had been taking Zoloft and other SSRI antidepressants.

• Alex Kim, age 13, hung himself shortly after his Lexapro prescription had been doubled.

• Diane Routhier was prescribed Welbutrin for gallstone problems. Six days later, after suffering many adverse effects of the drug, she shot herself.

• Billy Willkomm, an accomplished wrestler and a University of Florida student, was prescribed Prozac at the age of 17. His family found him dead of suicide – hanging from a tall ladder at the family's Gulf Shore Boulevard home in July 2002.

• Kara Jaye Anne Fuller-Otter, age 12, was on Paxil when she hung herself from a hook in her closet. Kara's parents said ".... the damn doctor wouldn't take her off it and I asked him to when we went in on the second visit. I told him I thought she was having some sort of reaction to Paxil...")

• Gareth Christian, Vancouver, age 18, was on Paxil when he committed suicide in 2002, (Gareth's father could not accept his son's death and killed himself.)

• Julie Woodward, age 17, was on Zoloft when she hung herself in her family's detached garage.

• Matthew Miller was 13 when he saw a psychiatrist because he was having difficulty at school. The psychiatrist gave him samples of Zoloft. Seven days later his mother found him dead, hanging by a belt from a laundry hook in his closet.

• Kurt Danysh, age 18, and on Prozac, killed his father with a shotgun. He is now behind prison bars, and writes letters, trying to warn the world that SSRI drugs can kill.

• Woody __, age 37, committed suicide while in his 5th week of taking Zoloft. Shortly before his death his physician suggested doubling the dose of the drug. He had seen his physician only for insomnia. He had never been depressed, nor did he have any history of any mental illness symptoms.

• A boy from Houston, age 10, shot and killed his father after his Prozac dosage was increased.

• Hammad Memon, age 15, shot and killed a fellow middle school student. He had been diagnosed with ADHD and depression and was taking Zoloft and "other drugs for the conditions."

• Matti Saari, a 22-year-old culinary student, shot and killed 9 students and a teacher, and wounded another student, before killing himself. Saari was taking an SSRI and a benzodiazapine.

• Steven Kazmierczak, age 27, shot and killed five people and wounded 21 others before killing himself in a Northern Illinois University auditorium. According to his girlfriend, he had recently been taking Prozac, Xanax and Ambien. Toxicology results showed that he still had trace amounts of Xanax in his system.

• Finnish gunman Pekka-Eric Auvinen, age 18, had been taking antidepressants before he killed eight people and wounded a dozen more at Jokela High School – then he committed suicide.

• Asa Coon from Cleveland, age 14, shot and wounded four before taking his own life. Court records show Coon was on Trazodone.

• Jon Romano, age 16, on medication for depression, fired a shotgun at a teacher in his New York high school."

Full article is here: *http://www.naturalnews.com/ 039752_mass_shootings_psychiatric_drugs_antidepressants.html#ixzz3VqGdo8rF*

It was also confirmed that Aurora "Batman" shooter James Holmes was taking *Sertraline* and *Clonazepam*.

And now that we've seen that these drugs cause batshit crazy behavior, let's look at some of the other side effects. This is from *WebMD.com*:

"Call 911 or other emergency services right away if you have:

Trouble breathing.
Swelling of your face, lips, tongue, or throat.

Call your doctor if you have:

Hives.
Thoughts of suicide.
Agitation and restlessness.
Seizures.
Fast heartbeat.
Nausea and vomiting.

Common side effects of this medicine include:

Loss of sexual desire or ability.
Irritability.
Trouble sleeping or drowsiness.
Headache.
Changes in appetite.

FDA advisories. The U.S. Food and Drug Administration (FDA) has issued:

An advisory on antidepressant medicines and the risk of suicide. Talk with your doctor about these possible side effects and the warning signs of suicide.

A warning about taking triptans, used for headaches, with SSRIs (selective serotonin reuptake inhibitors) or SNRIs (selective serotonin/norepinephrine reuptake inhibitors). Taking these medicines together can cause a very rare but serious condition called serotonin syndrome."

Full article is here: *http://www.webmd.com/depression/selective-serotonin-reuptake-inhibitors-ssris-for-depression*

I cannot express myself clearly enough on this issue. Mere words are not enough. Remember, these are *supposed to be* "medicines" that *promote mental/pschological wellbeing*! Can we get just a little bit more ridiculous? With all of this evidence that they clearly *do not* promote mental/pschological well being, with all of this evidence that they actually *promote the exact opposite* in far, far too many cases, wouldn't it be safe to say that these drugs should be pulled from the market? Anyone with any common sense can simply look at the facts and derive that conclusion! It's not rocket science. But of course the powers that be do not see it that way. They think that issuing an official "Black Box Warning" is good enough, and then they allow business as usual, never mind all of the school shootings, etc. because what this is *really* all about is making money for the drug companies, nothing more! The FDA has no intention of removing these drugs from the market, because they are working in support of the drug companies and looking out for their profit margins. The idea that the FDA looks out for the safety of the people is a bullshit lie, plain and simple. *Clearly* these drugs are dangerous beyond description and *clearly* they should not be used under any circumstances! But the FDA allows them to be prescribed and sold at alarming rates. *Harvard Medical School's* website has this to say about it:

"Remember when the best-selling book Listening to Prozac came out almost 20 years ago?

Now Americans aren't just reading about Prozac. They are taking it and other antidepressants (Celexa, Effexor, Paxil, Zoloft, to name just a few) in astounding numbers.

According to a report released yesterday by the National Center for Health Statistics (NCHS), the rate of antidepressant use in this country among teens and adults (people ages 12 and older) increased by almost 400% between 1988–1994 and 2005–2008.

The federal government's health statisticians figure that about one in every 10 Americans takes an antidepressant. And by their reckoning, antidepressants were the third most common prescription medication taken by Americans in 2005–2008, the latest period during which the National Health and Nutrition Examination Survey (NHANES) collected data on prescription drug use."

Full article is here: *http://www.health.harvard.edu/blog/astounding-increase-in-antidepressant-use-by-americans-201110203624*

And from *MedScape.com*:

"...*the antipsychotic aripiprazole (Abilify, Otsuka Pharmaceutical) had the highest sales, at nearly $6.5 billion*, according to a new report from research firm IMS Health on the top 100 selling drugs in the United States."

Full article is here: *http://www.medscape.com/viewarticle/820011*

"Antipsychotic"? Ha! Who are they fooling? Wait, never mind.

Obviously they're fooling millions of gullible people. One look at their sales records makes that obvious. Again, *"Beam me up Scotty, there's no intelligent life on this planet."* Who keeps these drug dealers in business? Ignorant people do. People who are willing to comply with their "doctor", the sales reps for Big Pharma, that's who! And with profits like that who cares about safety? Not the FDA! They work for the drug companies, get it? One hand washes the other, get it? Money talks, bullshit walks, get it? Corruption rules, get it? God Bless America, get it? The land of profits first and people last, get it? Drugs are good for you, get it? They create "health", get it? Sure, people go apeshit and shoot up schools with sub-machine guns, but hey, who cares? Not us! We like our money, thanks very much.

Can you tell I'm a little bit perturbed by all of this? That's an understatement. I am *very upset* by all of this, and this book is upsetting for me to write, but it has to be written for humanity's sake. The more people who read this and wake up to the *corruption* of the *drug pushers* and wake up to the *reality* of safe and natural treatments for their ailments, the better! Humanity must awaken and remove these scumbags from power. If everyone grew their own herbs and used it as medicine, how much power would the drug pushers have? Not much. *Not any!* Their party would be over. If everyone did what I am doing and acted as their own naturopathic physician, how powerful would the drug paradigm be? The goal here is to *educate the people* and *raise consciousness* for the good of humanity.

Herbs for depression? Well yes, but it goes beyond that. Holistic medicine emphasizes finding the *root cause* of problems. We must analyze our lifestyles, our diets, our surroundings, our thinking processes, and everything else. If your lifestyle includes ingesting chemicals into your body on a daily basis, for example diet soda (which contains *aspartame*, an addictive, cancer causing neurotoxin which causes depression and is associated with 92 different health issues; see ***Appendix C*** for more info) and other "foods" that people consume that are loaded down with chemicals, then that needs to be considered. If you're exposed to lots of EMF's at work, exposed to environmental toxins, sit in front of a computer every day, or whatever, then those things need to be considered as well. Do you have positive or negative thinking habits? Is the glass half full or half empty? All of these things are capable of contributing to depression and health problems.

I once read about a woman who had been severely depressed for decades, 30+ years, in and out of mental institutions, jail, etc. because she couldn't manage her moods, they had complete control of her. Eventually she got a tip from someone who suggested she have her mercury fillings removed and just like that, within a few days of removing them her depression "magically" disappeared. That's all it took. And that's my point. She was subjected to the mainstream drug pushing paradigm for many years, on and off of various drugs, in and out of various institutions, but they had no answers because they don't even look for the *root cause* of the problem, **they just drug people**.

My point is that there are numerous factors involved in every health issue. There is a *cause*, sometimes it's a direct *cause*, sometimes it's a more compound issue or more complex *cause*, but ultimately there is a *cause*, and that is the goal of holistic medicine practitioners as opposed to just providing drugs (or even herbs) and then calling it good. The *cause* has to be addressed, that's the main goal.

Drugs are commonly prescribed for symptom relief but they typically only cause new symptoms while merely putting a mask on the old ones. That's a lousy treatment method. Holistic medicine practitioners have much more than that in mind when they use herbs and supplements. They aren't just looking to mask symptoms. Herbs and supplements aren't replacements for drugs, not in the long run. Herbs *do* address symptoms, but in a safe and natural way, and they also provide nutrition and serve as *preventatives*. Drugs do no such thing. Deficiencies cause disease. In the long run herbs provide nutritional support and assist in balancing the body's system, eliminating health problems naturally. This certainly makes a lot more sense that popping a drug full of toxic chemicals to mask a symptom wouldn't you say? It's called being wise and rejecting harmful methods of so-called "health care".

The other goal, aside from finding the cause of the problem, is to address all *deficiencies*, because when your body has all of the nutrients that it requires you'll feel better in general and you won't get sick nearly as much. And that is why, again, I take three large handfuls of supplements and herbs every day. My goal is to fortify my nutrients and address all *deficiencies*, providing myself with *preventative medicine.*

When it comes to depression you can be assured that diet is very commonly a factor. Lousy eating and nutritional habits create people who simply don't feel good. Why don't you feel good? Because you're not taking proper care of your body. When you don't give your body proper nutrition it complains. One of the "side effects" of lousy diet and nutrition habits is depression. Others include low energy, headaches, water retention, gout (remember what I said about gout?), diabetes, high lipids, high blood pressure (remember what I said about low carb diets?), etc. *Improper eating habits* and *lack of proper nutrition* are *huge factors* when it comes to *all aspects* of health. If you eat pizza, french fries and Coca-Cola for lunch and dinner seven days a week, with coffee and donuts in the morning for breakfast, how do you suspect you'll feel as a result of a diet like that? If you're not feeling well physically do you think you'll feel well mentally? It all goes together. You can't just eat junk food and chemicals and then pop an "antidepressant" full of *yet more chemicals* and call it good. You need to accept personal responsibility for your mental and physical health. Does this make sense to you? I certainly hope so, and I also hope that you're realizing now that most cases of depression are in fact preventable and repairable without drugs, simply by addressing lifestyle factors, diet and nutritional deficiencies. The following deficiencies can lead to symptoms of depression:

- Biotin
- Chromium
- Folic Acid
- GABA
- Low blood sugar (hypoglycemia)
- Niacin
- Omega-3 Fatty Acids
- Pantothenic Acid
- Riboflavin
- S-adenosyl-methionine (SAM-e)
- Selenium
- Thiamine
- Thyroid deficiency (hypothyroidism)
- Trace Minerals
- Vitamin B6
- Vitamin B12
- Vitamin C

- Vitamin D
- Zinc
+ others!

Once again, *deficiencies* cause illness, in this case a *mental* illness called depression. And again, I take three large handfuls of supplements a day because they keep the "doctor" away! Proper nutrition can save you from dealing with many health problems, and if you think that you can get all of the nutrients that your body requires from your food, think again! Not possible! Taking supplements is *mandatory*, especially in the day and age of chemical and genetically modified "food" and microwave ovens where virtually all of the nutritional value is destroyed!

The general idea behind SSRI (selective serotonin reuptake inhibitors) drugs is that they assist in inhibiting the reuptake of serotonin at the nerve endings in the brain, the result being more serotonin binding to the receptor sites transmitting a more powerful serotonin signal. Serotonin, you see, is a very powerful neurotransmitter acting as the brain's own natural anti-depressant and tranquilizer. Low levels of serotonin do indeed lead to depression and many other conditions.

Not only does serotonin act as an antidepressant and tranquilizer, it also regulates the activity of many other neurotransmitters. But the problem with SSRI drugs is their severe side effects. Most people who take these drugs, if they're not experiencing violent reactions to these drugs, are at minimum experiencing at least *some* side effects. According to Dr. Michael Murray N.D. in his book *What the Drug Companies Won't Tell You and Your Doctor Doesn't Know* roughly 20% of people experience nausea; 20% experience headaches; 15% anxiety and nervousness; 14% insomnia; 12% drowsiness; 12% diarrhea; 9.5% dry mouth; 8% sweating and tremor; and 3% rash. He also says that many of his patients experienced rapid weight gain due to using these drugs because they "alter an area of the brain that regulates both serotonin levels and utilization of *glucose*" intensifying hunger and cravings.

There is no argument that low serotonin levels lead to depression and that raising those levels can relieve symptoms, but the controversy lies in how to achieve that goal. People with no common sense argue that these drugs are ok, but what do *you* now think, considering what I have shown you so far concerning the severe side effects and violent behaviors associated with these drugs? Holistic health practitioners have other ideas about how to raise serotonin levels *naturally* and *without those very negative side effects.*

There are numerous herbs and supplements which increase serotonin levels and act as tranquilizers to the nervous system. I'll start by listing the ones that specifically either raise or aid serotonin levels and/or functionality:

- 5-Hydroxytriptophan ("5-HTP" a natural precursor to serotonin)
- Gingko Biloba
- Omega-3 Fatty Acids (Fish Oil)
- SAM-e
- St. John's Wort

In an article entitled *"5-HTP (5-Hydroxytryptophan) vs. Prozac (SSRIs)"* by Ward Dean, M.D., James South, M.A. and Jim English they state:

"Fortunately, a safe, natural and effective alternative...has been researched for over 30 years. This substance, L-5-Hydroxytryptophan (5-HTP)..is extracted from the seeds of the Griffonia plant. In one study, the antidepressant effects of 5-HTP were compared with fluvoxamine, a prescription Prozac-like drug used in Europe. The 5-HTP patients showed slightly better treatment response than the fluvoxamine group, yet had significantly fewer and less severe side effects. The researchers note: 'Regarding tolerance and safety, however, 5-HTP proved superior to fluvoxamine as was apparent from a marked difference in severity of untoward side effects between the two compounds. The study presented here ...strongly confirm[s] the efficacy of 5-HTP as an antidepressant.'

"The many successful published studies using 5-HTP show that 5-HTP, by naturally elevating brain serotonin, can alleviate the serotonin-deficiency syndrome without any help from SSRI drugs. Yet the success of SSRI drugs is crucially dependent upon the brain producing adequate serotonin (from either tryptophan or 5-HTP), and that brain serotonin production is the controlling or rate-limiting variable underlying the apparent success of SSRIs. It appears that the more logical and economically sound choice to alleviate conditions that result from the serotonin deficiency syndrome is 5-HTP, the immediate precursor of the deficient substance."

Full article is here: *http://www.crossroadsinitiative.com/ library_article/725/5_htp_vs._prozac_jim_english.html*

As you can see above, a natural substance extracted from Griffonia plant seeds (5-HTP) is very effective, *more effective*, for depression than drugs, and it doesn't cause suicidal thoughts or mass shootings! Gee whiz Wally, what a concept!

The following herbs/supplements address the nervous system and they do a *fine job* of it too:

- Black Currant Oil

- Cannabis ("Marijuana")
- Chamomile
- Chinese Club Moss
- Feverfew
- Fennel Seed
- Hops
- Inositol
- Kava Kava
- Lecithin
- Lobelia
- Marshmallow Root
- Passion Flower
- Valerian Root
- White Willow

Clearly, unless one has a very severe case of chronic depression, drugs are totally unnecessary. By looking at the comparison between 5-HTP and the "Prozac-like drug" we can see that 5-HTP was a more beneficial treatment on every level. And when you combine that with other factors such as diet, environmental toxins, and others, the need for these drugs becomes virtually null and void. In rare cases where people are committed to institutions these drugs might be warranted, but even then, we need to remember that mainstream "medicine" does nothing to try and address the **root cause** of the problem. Their methods are *drugs first* with everything else either taking secondary priority or no priority at all, which is, of course, and act in criminal negligence and a crime against humanity. Clearly, the paradigm must change!

Various Common Ailments

Before I finish up this section on my personal health history and get to the heavy duty corruption of the *American Medical Association* and Big Pharma in part two, I'd like to address some other minor ailments that have afflicted me from time to time.

Psoriasis/Rash/Skin Problems

Due to my hypothyroidism I had some very annoying skin problems. I had scalp psoriasis so bad that when I scratched my head it was a major snow storm! I had patches on my head the size of quarters and patches on my hips and lower middle back as well. I battled this for a long time and tried seemingly everything. Nothing worked.

One night while casually searching YouTube I stumbled upon a home-made video by a middle aged woman who was praising a product for curing her psoriasis. I took it with a grain of salt but I thought I'd watch just in case. She said that she had terrible psoriasis for 20+ years so bad that she was embarrassed to shake hands with people because she had it on her hands too, and she said that when she tried this product her psoriasis magically disappeared almost immediately. I was still a bit skeptical due to trying so many things and failing every time, but I had nothing to lose, so I went out and got the product she endorsed.

When I started this book I told myself that I wouldn't endorse any products. I don't want this book to be a commercial for various products, which is why I don't mention brand names, only various herbs and supplements, but in this case I will make an exception to that rule because the lady very specifically mentioned this product and if you, the reader, have psoriasis I want you to know what the product is. It is called *DOO GROW Stimulating Growth Oil* and it contains a blend of various herbs and natural oils:

- Butyrospermum Parkii (Shea) Butter Extract
- Calendula Officinalis Flower Extract
- Carthamus Tinctorius (Safflower) Seed Oil
- Chamomilla Recutita (Matricaria) Extract
- Equisetum Hyemale Extract
- Humulus Lupulus (Hops) Extract

- Hydrastis Canadensis (Golden Seal) Extract
- Limanthes Alba (Meadowfoam) Seed Oil
- Lawsonia Inermis (Henna) Extract
- Paraffinum Liquidum (Mineral Oil)
- Prunus Amygdalus Dulcis (Sweet Almond) Oil
- Prunus Serotina (Wild Cherry) Bark Extract
- Quillaja Saponaria Bark Extract
- Triticum Vulgare (Wheat) Germ Oil
- Zea Mays (Corn) Oil

I was excited when I saw the lady's video and I ran out and got some *Doo Grow* immediately. Within a couple of days I noticed a difference and within a week my psoriasis was completely gone, which is yet more evidence that herbs are superior to drugs. I'd tried "medicated" shampoo, ointments, etc and nothing worked, but when I used a natural blend of herbs my psoriasis was cured. It did come back months after I discontinued using the product, so I stocked up on it and I've been using it whenever I feel I need to, but I've noticed that because of taking natural desiccated thyroid and ridding myself of hypothyroidism symptoms my skin problems have cleared up significantly and I rarely need to use skin treatments any more.

I've also had rashes/fungus in various spots. Since I've taken up herbalism I've learned of various herbs that work miracles on skin. Aside from the herbs mentioned above in *Doo Grow* there are:

- Aloe Vera
- Burdock Root
- Chamomile Flowers
- Coconut Oil
- Comfrey Root
- Gotu Kola
- Green Tea
- Horsetail
- Lavender
- Lemongrass
- Licorice Root
- Oregon Grape Root
- Peppermint
- Pomegranate
- St. John's Wort
- Tea Tree Oil
+ more!

<u>Conjunctivitis (Pinkeye)</u>

We've all had pinkeye before right? If you haven't you're lucky. The last time for me was an extremely aggravating experience. I was like most people, I didn't know how to handle the problem on my own. There were no over the counter eye drops that would work (as far as I knew) because it was a bacterial infection, but I knew that there were "special" antibiotic eye drops that I could get if I went to a "doctor" so I pursued that route. I was given a prescription for *Vigamox* antibiotic eyedrops. I was happy until I went to the pharmacy! I had no insurance at the time you see. They said that they had no "generic" brand and the price (at that time) was, if I remember correctly, about $60.00. Keep in mind that I was only given a teeny tiny little bottle containing 3 ml (milliliters) of eye drops. Let's put this into terms you can understand. For $60.00 I was given about **one tenth** of an **ounce** of solution! I just looked on WalMart's bargain pharmacy website again, and the price on this item currently (March, 2015) is $143.33 "with free coupon"! *Now* do all of my readers understand my frustration? How much do you think it costs to produce a tiny bottle, about a *tenth of an ounce*, of solution like that? My guess is about three cents! Probably less than that! Yes, I was pissed! (As a side note, it is a known *fact* that drug companies sometimes mark up their prices by as much as *2000%*. That's **two thousand percent**!)

At the time I was ignorant to the alternative routes, so I slammed the money on the counter, took my eye drops and left with steam coming out of my ears. This is a perfect example of the *sheer greed and corruption of the pharmaceutical industry* taking advantage of the common people and sodomizing them without the benefit of a lubricant!

Here I am about three years later and now *I know all about herbs*. I now know how to make eye drops that will knock out an eye infection for a mere couple of bucks! There is one herb in particular that works best for this and it is called *Eyebright* (the next best one would be *Goldenseal*). All you have to do is boil them in distilled water, strain off the herbs and let it cool. Tada! You have an antibiotic eyewash and a cure for pinkeye! Even if you're not using bulk herb and making it yourself it's still very inexpensive. For about $10.00 you can get a two ounce bottle of *Eyebright* tincture at any health food store, and when you use it all you have to do is put five drops into an ounce of boiled, distilled water, let it cool and then flush your eyes with it or use it as eyedrops. Pretty simple!

Drug companies, if you're reading, I have *two middle fingers* flying high in the air just for you! Never again will I pay for your overpriced eye drops!

Common Cold/Flu

As I said earlier, due to my daily intake of colloidal silver I haven't been sick much in the last five years, but I have managed to get a few colds due to inhalation of cold air during the winter. There was only one day where I was too ill to work in five years, and that was because I had an upper respiratory infection. At that point I was still fairly new to herbalism, but I was determined not to use any drugs stronger than *Tylenol*, so I did a little bit of research and took a trip to the health food store. I purchased a blend of *Echinacea* with *Goldenseal*, started taking it three times daily, and within one day I was well enough to work again.

Echinacea is a very powerful immune system stimulator, one of the very best, as well as a blood purifying agent. *Goldenseal* is also a very potent blood purifier, and a powerful expectorant that clears mucus from the upper respiratory and nasal areas. Combining these two herbs makes for a very powerful cold remedy.

There are, of course, many other methods of dealing with common colds. The antibiotic herbs listed in the MRSA section can be used with good results and so can these:

- Andrographis (enhances immune system, clears mucus)
- Astragalus (enhances immune system)
- Boneset (reduces fevers)
- Cat's Claw (eases cold symptoms)
- Elderberry (addresses upper respiratory and relieves headaches, makes a great tea!)
- Eucalyptus (relieves congestion, works great in vaporizers)
- Feverfew (reduces fevers, relieves headaches especially migraines)
- Ginger Root (enhances immune system, relieves headaches, reduces fever, tea is a great way to take this herb, drink lots!)
- Hyssop (clears mucus, antiviral)
- Mullien (cough suppressant)

- Olive Leaf Extract (spraying the tincture onto sore throats is very effective)
- Pelargonium Sidoides (relieves acute bronchitis)
- Red Clover (detoxification of the lymph system)
- Sage (antibacterial, relieves sore throat, clears mucus, reduces fever, reduces sweating)
- Tea Tree Oil (three drops in some warm water as a gargle for sore throats)
- Thyme (enhances immune system, antibacterial, cough suppressant)
- White Willow Bark Extract (reduces fevers, relieves headaches)
- Wild Cherry Bark (relieves cough)

I was also taking *White Willow Bark Extract,* which contains *Salicin,* the main ingredient in aspirin, for the **headache**: There are many herbs that work great for headaches and migraines. Other than *White Willow* there are:

- 5-HTP
- Bay Leaf
- Butterbur
- Cayenne
- Elderberry
- Eucalyptus
- Feverfew
- Ginger Root (drink Ginger Root Tea!)
- Gingko Biloba
- Grape Seed Extract
- Meadowsweet (also contains salicin)
- MSM
- Passionflower
- Peppermint
- Pine Bark Extract
- Valerian Root

And if you're nauseated, feeling like you have to hurl, there's nothing that works better than *Ginger Root Tea.* Simply boil some ginger root in some water and drink up!

Many common over-the-counter drugs have harmful side effects; for example aspirin can cause ulcers, destroy the lining of the stomach and cause internal bleeding. *Tylenol* and other similar drugs are very hard on liver function. A 2015 article from *GreenMedInfo.com* entitled *"Ibuprofen Kills Thousands Each Year, So What Is The Alternative?"* states:

"A recent Reuters' article opened with the following stunning sentence:

'Long-term high-dose use of painkillers such as ibuprofen or diclofenac is 'equally hazardous' in terms of heart attack risk as use of the drug Vioxx, which was withdrawn due to its potential dangers, researchers said.'

The 2004 Vioxx recall, as you may remember, was spurred by the nearly 30,000 excess cases of heart attacks and sudden cardiac deaths caused by the drug between 1999-2003. Despite the fact that scientific research had accumulated as early as 2000 linking Vioxx to increased heart attacks and strokes, the drug's manufacturer Merck, and the FDA, remained silent as the death toll steadily increased."

Full article is here: *http://www.greenmedinfo.com/blog/ibuprofen-kills-more-pain-so-what-alternatives*

They might clear up your cold or cure your headache, but not any better than the safe and natural supplements mentioned above. Why use drugs when the health food store has natural alternatives that work great? Next time you feel a cold coming on, go get some *Echinacea* with *Goldenseal* and some *White Willow Bark Extract*. And don't forget about *Colloidal Silver* either! They work great!

Part Two:
The Medical Mafia Exposed

In **Part One** you saw my personal health history and the various medical problems that I've had to deal with in my life so far. You saw that I chose to branch off and deal with those problems on my own due to the sheer incompetence of the mainstream medical establishment. You saw the research that I did on natural alternatives to drugs and you saw that I was successful in taking better care of myself by taking the self-educated naturopathic route than by allowing my care to be in the hands of the drug pushing "health care" system. You also saw many examples of criminal negligence and corruption in the pharmaceutical and medical industries; lies about cholesterol to sell their drugs, the unnecessary prescribing of millions of rounds of antibiotics, the suppression of the cure for MRSA in the form of colloidal silver and various other effective treatments for MRSA, numerous examples of deadly toxic drugs that are routinely prescribed like candy and are totally and completely unnecessary, and of course, you saw the alternatives to these drugs which are every bit as effective minus the toxicity.

In **Part Two** I'll be discussing things that I have never personally had to deal with, yet are urgently important. I'll be presenting information here that is very upsetting, especially if you, like me, have relatives that have passed away from AIDS and cancer.

You'll see that the "HIV causes AIDS" theory is not only unproven, it's easily debunked. HIV doesn't cause AIDS, the so-called "treatments" for HIV+ people do. Please don't write me off as a nutjob/conspiracy theorist until you've read the HIV/AIDS section. Learn something please! When you understand just how corrupt these people are, it makes a lot more sense!

You'll also see that there are not one, but *numerous* cures for cancer. **Proven cures**. And you'll see that doctors who are successful at curing cancers are *continually harassed and threatened by the FDA*. What's the official excuse from the FDA concerning their harassment of doctors who cure cancer? They say that they're using "unapproved methods", and of course, they're *not going to approve* any of those methods because they can't be patented, and because current cancer "treatments" rake them in billions upon billions of dollars in profits annually! If it cuts into their profits, they won't approve it! Very simple, yet very true!

I'll be discussing the drugging of children and the *bullshit excuses* that are used to put them on drugs like *Ritalin*, which affects the brain in exactly the same manner as cocaine.

I'll also be discussing not only childhood vaccines, but vaccines in general, and the lies perpetuated by the entire system concerning those vaccines. I'll show you the ingredients in vaccines and I'll show you why they kill and maim, cause autism, sudden infant death syndrome and destroy the immune system as opposed to what they're claimed to do, "prevent disease".

Part Two is the heaviest part of the book by a long shot. This information is upsetting to read, and even more upsetting for me to write, but again, for humanity's sake the truth must be put forward so that we, as a collective whole can evolve, grow and wise up, taking the power away from the dark forces in control of our medical system. *They must be stopped!*

Before I proceed I'd like to give you a little history lesson:

In 1910 John D. Rockefeller had a goal in life. He wanted to dominate the world's pharmaceutical market. In order to get started with the pharmaceuticals his company (*Standard Oil of New Jersey*) purchased a controlling interest in *I.G. Farben*, a German drug/chemical company. Rockefeller then hired a man named Abraham Flexner to "assess" the medical schools and write a biased report to the *Carnegie Foundation* entitled *"Medical Education in the United States and Canada"* now commonly known as the *"Flexner Report"*. The report recommended, under the guise of "protection of the common people", making courses in pharmacology stronger, as well as the addition of research departments at the schools. His recommendation was sold to the public as something that was necessary in order to make their medical system more efficient, and conveniently it was exactly what Rockefeller wanted. The report also suggested that everything else (natural methods) were all pseudoscience and quackery. In other words, they were rigging it so that drugs would be the norm, and all competition would be ridiculed.

The public bought into his fake report hook, line and sinker, and the result was, of course, public backing and support, exactly what Rockefeller wanted and had planned all along. He then started funding *only* the schools that taught what he wanted; *drug therapy.* In order to continue receiving funding the schools had to continue to teach what Rockefeller wanted and any school that didn't comply *got their funding cut off,* which resulted in medical schools being geared towards drugs first and foremost.

In 1913 the *American Medical Association* (AMA) established a *Propaganda Department* which was designed for the purpose of attacking any and all non-drug treatments and anyone who prescribed them.

> "Soon after the medical monopoly was formed, it began to push its agenda of destroying all competition. A well organized and well-funded nationwide purge of all non-MD's was undertaken. Over the course of the first half of the 20th century this medical monopoly managed to shut down over 40 medical schools. Their idea was to keep the number of doctors low in order to keep fees up. After WWII the medical monopoly started rigidly controlling how many of each medical specialty it would allow to be trained. The medical monopoly also managed to outlaw or marginalize over 70 healthcare professions. 'Protection of the healthcare customer' was, as always, the rationale for this power grab. Whether the object of destruction by the medical monopoly be homeopaths, midwives, chiropractors, on internet prescribers, the purge is conducted in the same manner. No scientific proof or research data is offered to discredit these practitioners. The entire approach is one of character assassination."

> - Dr. Henry Jones

Over 10,000 herbalists were out of business by 1925. Over 1500 chiropractors were prosecuted for practicing "quackery" by 1940. Between 1900 and 1922 homeopathic schools were reduced down from 22 existing schools to 2. By 1950 there were none left. "Training" from the Flexner approved medical "schools" were the only way people could practice. Despite the legitimacy of these other practices, they were forced out by the powers that be which eventually became Big Pharma.

Eventually the AMA became the national accrediting agency for medical schools, pushing its bias towards drug therapy even further. And the rest is history, as they say. That is how the "drug paradigm" and Big Pharma was born, and that is how the suppression of proven and effective natural (but **not patentable**) treatments got started. No money to be made? It cuts into our profits? Well then, let's ridicule it and force it out of existence!

Interestingly, the *American Medical Association* is *not* a government entity, it's a *private corporation,* a labor union. And like all labor unions, it has mafia bosses, hence the term "Medical

Mafia". And, as with all corporations, their motto should appropriately be "profits first, people last". The government does little to regulate them because the Rockefellers are one of the families that also own and control the *"Federal Reserve"* banking cartel (*also a private business!*) which just happens to control the USA's money supply, its government and its politicians. *Again,* before you accuse me of being a nutjob/conspiracy theorist I advise you to watch a film called *The Money Masters: How International Bankers Gained Control of America* on *YouTube.com* and visit the website at *TheMoneyMasters.com*. I also advise you to read my first book entitled *LOVE - EVOLVE - TRANSCEND: Building a Spiritual Culture on the Planet Earth* which gives more info on that subject as well.

ADHD Is a Fictitious Disorder

ADHD is a myth, a fictitious disease invented and perpetuated by drug companies in order to sell more drugs. "Whoa! Wait just a minute Mr. Dyer! What are you, some kind of a conspiracy theorist? Where's your tin foil hat?"

OK, well then, let's have a look at the following article from *NaturalNews.com*'s website entitled *"Before his death, father of ADHD admitted it was a fictitious disease"*:

"On his death bed, this psychiatrist and autism pioneer admitted that ADHD is essentially a 'fictitious disease,' which means that millions of young children today are being needlessly prescribed severe mind-altering drugs that will set them up for a life of drug addiction and failure.

ADHD was merely a theory developed by Eisenberg. It was never actually proven to exist as a verifiable disease, despite the fact that Eisenberg and many others profited handsomely from its widespread diagnosis. And modern psychiatry continues to profit as well, helping also to fill the coffers of the pharmaceutical industry by getting children addicted early to dangerous psychostimulant drugs like Ritalin (methylphenidate) and Adderall (amphetamine, dextroamphetamine mixed salts).

The purpose all along for pathologizing ADHD symptoms, of course, was to generate more profits for the drug industry. According to the citizen watchdog group Citizens Commission on Human Rights International (CCHRI), roughly 20 million American children today are taking dangerous, but expensive, psychiatric drugs for made-up behavioral conditions like ADHD. And another one million or so children have been blatantly and admittedly misdiagnosed with phony behavioral conditions for which psychiatric medications are being prescribed.

'Remember, there are two ways drug companies can make money: Invent new drugs, and invent new diseases already invented drugs can treat,' writes Dr. Jay Parkinson, M.D., M.P.H., about the fake disease-creation industry. 'In the past decade or so, Big Pharma has created no less than 10 new novel drugs per year,' he adds."

Full article is here: *http://www.naturalnews.com/ 040938_adhd_fictitious_disease_psychiatry.html#ixzz3WTyWZemV*

As you can clearly see, I'm not just making things up. Even the "father of ADHD," the man who *invented* the term, said *"ADHD is a prime example of a fictitious disease."* - Leon Eisenberg.

In order to make my point even more clear, let's have a look at the 18 standard so-called "symptoms" of ADHD, keeping in mind that **only 5** of these are required to be officially diagnosed with ADHD:

- Fails to pay close attention to details
- Has difficulty sustaining attention in tasks
- Does not seem to listen when spoken to directly
- Does not follow through on instructions

- Has difficulty organizing tasks/activities
- Avoids or dislikes tasks requiring sustained mental effort
- Loses things necessary for specific tasks
- Easily distracted by external stimuli
- Forgetful in daily activities
- Fidgets with hands/feet
- Leaves seat in situations where remaining seated is expected
- Runs about when inappropriate to do so
- Has difficulty engaging in leisure activities quietly
- Often on the go or acts as if driven by a motor
- Talks excessively
- Blurts out answers
- Has difficulty awaiting turns
- Interrupts or intrudes on others

Source: *ADHD Does Not Exist: The Truth About Attention Deficit and Hyperactivity Disorder* by Richard Saul

So can we *get real* for just a second please!? Go take another look at those so-called "symptoms". No, go ahead, I'll wait....

Now, how many of those symptoms are *abnormal* for children? Make a list! Go ahead, go do it, I'll keep waiting...

Uh huh. Just as I thought. You couldn't find *one* example in that list that doesn't define a *normal child*! How many children do you know who fit **less than 5** of those so-called "symptoms"? I personally don't know any! *Every child alive* can easily be described by 5 of the items on that list with no problems whatsoever. When I was a kid they called all of those things *"being a kid"*. Admit it! There is no *real definition* of what ADHD is, the "symptoms" are so vague that it could fit *any child*! ADHD is a *bullshit excuse* to sell drugs.

Kids are normally pretty energetic, hyper, talkative, etc. That's just part of being a kid. If you're experiencing a case that you believe to be abnormal then I'd like you to think about something else here. *Diet.* What is your child *eating*? So-called "foods" these days are typically loaded down with chemicals and sugars, especially the kind of foods that kids like to eat. What happens when we consume things like that? What happens when children eat a bunch of chemicals and sugar? Remember, their bodies and minds aren't fully developed yet. Their brains are still in the growing process. Public schools are notorious for feeding kids *cheap food.* School lunch plans are typically *very high in carbohydrates*. I remember my school lunches, they were pretty much *all carbs*. We've discussed carbs in this book quite a bit.

What's wrong with giving carbs to children? You should know by now if you've been paying attention. Carbs are *pure sugar.* Did you ever watch Beavis and Butthead? Do you remember the Great Cornholio who needs "TP" for his bunghole? Well, when you pump kids full of carbs (*sugars!*) that's what you get. You get little Cornholios running around, bouncing off the walls. So the school system pumps kids full of sugar (carbs) at lunch and then they send those kids back to classrooms where they're supposed to sit still and be quiet. When they're not sitting still and being quiet their teacher reports them, one thing leads to another and pretty soon they're diagnosed with ADHD and *being forced to take drugs.* For *what?* Because the school gave them *pure sugar* for lunch?

If you have a child who's abnormally "hyper" then take a look at what they *consume* every day. If their behavior is a problem put them on an "all natural" diet plan, keep the carbs low, and when they do eat carbs make sure they are carbs that are low on the glycemic index. The glycemic index indicates how quickly particular carbohydrates enter the bloodstream in the form of glucose (sugar). As I mentioned earlier, wheat products, those so-called "healthy" whole grains are *higher* on the glycemic index than *sugar itself.* If your child is hyper don't give them wheat products! Those products will only *contribute* to their hyperactivity. Google "glycemic index" to get an idea of what low glycemic foods are. Keep in mind that sugar itself is rated a 59 on the GI, therefore you need to stay away from foods that are *anywhere near* that number. A good rule of thumb would be to only give them foods that are rated a 30 or lower, preferably much lower, and to keep those foods as side dishes, not as main dishes. Their main staple foods should be foods that are *zero* in carbohydrates; meats, fish, chicken, green vegetables, salad, etc. Stay away from breads, potatoes and starchy vegetables. Those are high glycemic carbohydrates and will contribute to their hyperactivity!

Did I mention that schools are given financial incentives to "diagnose" kids with ADHD? In 1991 Federal Education Grants rules were changed. They granted $400.00 per student diagnosed with ADHD per year, resulting in a sudden spike in ADHD cases. Patti Johnson from the *Colorado State Board of Education* told the *US House of Representatives Subcommittee on Oversight and*

Investigations the following:

> "The IDEA legislation provided schools with $400 per year for each child in 'special education'. There followed a dramatic spike in the amount of methylphenidate consumed in the US. According to the DEA, the production and use of methylphenidate increased almost 6 fold between 1990 and 1995. In December 1999, the Los Angeles Times reported that tens of thousands of California's special education students were placed there not because they have a serious mental or emotional handicap, but because they were never taught to read properly. Reid Lyon, head of the federal government s research efforts into reading and writing told the Times, 'It is where children who weren't taught well go in many cases.'"

Also:

> "The so-called learning disorders have, sadly, become a way for financially strapped schools to make ends meet. In many states, schools have become authorized Medicaid providers and funds can be collected in behalf of a child labeled with one of the learning of behavioral disorders. This can be such a lucrative cash cow that in a letter dated October 8th, 1996, the Illinois State Board of Education strongly encouraged the superintendent of one of its districts to participate in Medicaid incentives. The letter stated that Illinois had received $72,500,000 in federal Medicaid money in 1996 and that Medicaid dollars have been used for a variety of non-medical purposes and that 'the potential for dollars is limitless.'"

So they create a convenient list of so-called "symptoms" that will fit *every child alive*, and then they provide financial incentives to schools to diagnose ADHD as much as possible. What a great plan! Talk about a great method of making drug profits! And who cares about the innocent children whose lives we're destroying, at least we're making money! There are currently *four million* innocent little kids on the powerful drug called *Ritalin* in the USA. *Ritalin* is the # 1 prescribed drug for ADHD. Did you happen to notice that one of the drugs often mentioned in the list of school shooters, one of the drugs that are often associated with criminally violent behavior is in fact *Ritalin*? Go back to the "Depression" section and take a look. That's because *Ritalin* is commonly prescribed as an antidepressant as well. The following is a list of side effects associated with *Ritalin* taken from *WebMD.com*:

> "The following side effects are associated with Ritalin:
>
> "Common side effects of Ritalin:
>
> - Fast Heartbeat
> - High Blood Pressure
> - Chronic Trouble Sleeping
> - Dry Mouth
> - Feel Like Throwing Up
> - Head Pain
> - Loss of Appetite
> - Nervous
> - Over Excitement

- Upper Abdominal Pain

"Infrequent side effects of Ritalin:

- Angina
- Chest Pain
- Decreased Blood Platelets
- Fever
- Hives
- Inflammation of Skin caused by an Allergy

- Involuntary Quivering
- Joint Pain
- Rash
- Reaction due to an Allergy
- Sinus Irritation and Congestion
- Voluntary Movement Difficulty
- Acute Infection of the Nose, Throat or Sinus
- Aggressive Behavior
- Cough
- Dizzy
- Drowsiness
- Excessive Sweating
- Stomach Cramps
- Throat Irritation
- Weight Loss

"Rare side effects of Ritalin:

- Abnormal Heart Rhythm
- Abnormal Liver Function Tests
- Anemia
- Blurred Vision
- Chronic Muscle Twitches or Movements
- Continued Painful Erection
- Decreased White Blood Cells
- Erythema Multiforme
- Failure to Grow
- Feeling Restless
- Fit
- Giant Hives
- Hallucination
- Heart Attack
- Hemorrhage in the Brain
- Inflammation of Blood Vessels that Carry Blood in the Brain
- Life Threatening Allergic Reaction
- Mental Disorder Resulting from Poisonous Agents
- Mental Disorder with Loss of Normal Personality & Reality
- Mood Changes
- Occasional Numbness, Prickling, or Tingling of Fingers and Toes
- Problems with Eyesight
- Seizures
- Skin Rash with Sloughing
- Stroke
- Worsening Symptoms of Tourette's Syndrome
- Altered Interest in Having Sexual Intercourse
- Confused
- Constriction of Blood Vessels of the Extremities
- Diarrhea

- Grinding of the Teeth
- Hair Loss
- Heart Throbbing or Pounding
- Hypertalkative
- Inflammation of the Nose
- Itching
- Migraine Headache
- Painful Periods
- Reversible Ischemic Neurological Defect
- Throwing Up

Full article is here: *http://www.webmd.com/drugs/2/drug-9475/ritalin-oral/details/list-sideeffects*

If you give your child this drug you're a negligent, abusive parent, plain and simple. If you didn't know what you were doing, if you were ignorant to the harm that you were doing to your child before you read this then you can no longer use ignorance as an excuse because *now you know*! Please review the list of so-called "side effects" of this drug again, and then try to get mad at me for stating the obvious. Only unfit parents give drugs like this to their children. It's called *child abuse*. And no, I don't care if your quack, drug pushing sales rep for Big Pharma "doctor" says it's ok. It's *not*!

"Ritalin is Very Similar to Cocaine

Ritalin and Cocaine are both Schedule II controlled Substances in the United States. They have similar chemical structures, stimulant effects, and addictive properties. They both work by increasing dopamine levels in the brain.

Ritalin and Cocaine block the natural reuptake process of dopamine at the synapse causing the synaptic cleft in between two neurons to be overfilled with dopamine.

Will taking Ritalin during childhood change how the brain develops?

The human brain continues to grow until around the age of thirty years old...It is common sense that crack-babies have had a bad start in life; and that mothers shouldn't take 'drugs' when they are carrying developing fetuses. It is also common knowledge that it is unhealthy for children to take cocaine. This is why the U.S. Government has made cocaine a Schedule II controlled substance. We all remember the government sponsored anti-drug commercials with an egg cracking in a pan, and an actor saying that 'this is your brain, and this is your brain on drugs.' We all know that it is against the law for a mother to give her ten year old a line of cocaine. If she gets caught doing so, she will have her children taken away by child welfare authorities, and then she will go to prison for at least fifteen years (triple the normal mandatory minimum sentence because the child was under eighteen). Then why does our government allow parents and doctors to put young children on stimulant ADHD drugs? Why isn't our government protecting us? Isn't that what the drug war was supposed to be about?"

Full article is here: *http://www.neurosoup.com/ritalin-the-real-gateway-drug/*

Ritalin is a very dangerous drug for *anybody*, and giving it to a child who isn't fully developed yet is again, child abuse. Instead of being lazy, drugging your children and destroying their lives, you should be actively involved with their nutrition habits as mentioned above, and if there's a genuine problem with behavior that goes beyond normal you should be working to isolate the *cause* of the problem. Masking and covering up symptoms with drugs can only mean one thing; *the problem remains* because as soon as you take the drug away the problem comes back! That's not a solution! And drugging children is *unacceptable*!

"If you stepped on a nail and the nail became embedded in your foot and caused an infection, you would expect the doctor to remove the nail. You would not expect the doctor to examine the extent of redness and the swelling of the foot, test the infected tissue for the exact type of infection occurring on the foot, clean the area, bandage it, and send you home with a prescription for antibiotics and orders to stay off the foot until it is healed, leaving the embedded nail in your foot. Imagine---the infection keep recurring because the source of the problem is still embedded in your body. The doctor simply prescribes stronger and stronger antibiotics to control the infection. And when that doesn't solve the infection problem, the doctor puts you on a long-term antibiotic treatment and declares you to be handicapped with a chronic infection that prevents you from walking on your foot. You cannot play sports or engage in other outside activities. In addition, you are exposed to the side effects of long-term antibiotic drug use, and the underlying problem of the nail in your foot will still be there when they take you off the medication.

This, in my opinion, is what we are doing to our children labeled with ADHD."

- **Dr. Mary Ann Block** in her book *No More Ritalin: Treating ADHD Without Drugs* page 60-61.

Dr. Block states in her book that the most common causes of abnormal behavior in children are:

- Dietary factors
- Allergies
- Hypoglycemia (low blood sugar level)
- Learning disabilities
- Hyperthyroidism (abnormally high metabolism)

"Doctors" typically do *nothing* to try and isolate those problems and almost *always* put the children on dangerous drugs like Ritalin instead! That is a crime against innocent children and will have a negative impact for generations to come. Please don't contribute to that by being an irresponsible parent! If you love your children don't abuse them with dangerous drugs! Use good judgment and common sense please!

Other drugs prescribed for ADHD include *Dexadrine, Cylert, Tofranil, Norpramin, Catapres, Prozac* and *Paxil*. If you go back to the section concerning so-called "antidepressant" drugs (the "Depression" section) you'll find that many of these drugs are used interchangeably as both antidepressants and treatments for ADHD. Please go back and review what I presented about those drugs concerning violent criminal behavior and then ask yourself if you should be giving those drugs to your children. Only a totally brain-dead, incompetent, negligent and unfit parent would willingly give those drugs to their child. Please wake up!

As you have seen above the "father of ADHD" admitted on his death bed that ADHD is a *"fictitious disease"*, it is "diagnosed" with a list of loose, vague symptoms that can and do *fit every child alive*, financial incentives are given to schools to "diagnose" ADHD and "doctors" rarely, if ever, look for the underlying causes of abnormal behavior in children, preferring to push dangerous drugs instead which, of course, makes Big Pharma more profits.

You've seen that dietary factors are the most common causes of abnormal behavior in children and now you know that modifying diet, looking for allergies and checking for real diseases like hyperthyroidism and hypoglycemia are much more appropriate methods of dealing with the problem as opposed to simply drugging your children into submission and turning them into zombies with toxic chemicals. Wake up parents, stop being dumb and stop abusing your children. Just because your "doctor" says it's ok doesn't mean it's ok. It's *not*!

Vaccines Kill, Maim and Spread Disease

Vaccines, a marvel of modern science. They're great. They stop people from getting sick. They wipe out diseases. They stopped polio. They protect babies from illness. They are one of modern medicine's greatest accomplishments and they are backed by scientific studies. Or so we're told...

But the blunt truth of the matter is that vaccines prevent *nothing*, period, and they cause serious injuries such as autism, sudden infant death, seizures and paralysis. They massively assist in *spreading* (not preventing) disease and they promote the very illnesses that they supposedly prevent. If the people of the world knew the truth, the vast majority would say "no thanks" to vaccines, especially if they understood that nutrition, vitamins, herbs and supplements build up the immune system enough to fight off almost any disease known to mankind, as opposed to what toxic vaccines do, which is *dramatically weaken the immune system*.

Sugar coating the truth is nothing I'm interested in doing, I'd rather just put it straight out there. So where shall I start? I guess I'll start by rattling off several examples of disease outbreaks in highly vaccinated populations:

- Measles outbreak in Texas, 1985. 99% were vaccinated. Only 1% were not.
 Source: *"New England Journal of Medicine"*; Volume 316; No. 13; pp. 771-774 (1987)

- Mumps outbreak in Iowa, 2006. 92% vaccinated. Only 8% were not.
Source: *Center for Disease Control*; MMWR; 55 (20); May 26, 2006; pp. 559-563

- Chickenpox outbreak in Oregon, 2004. 86% vaccinated. Only 14% were not.
Source: *"Pediatrics"*; Volume 113; No. 3; pp. 455-459 (2004)

- Pertussis outbreak in Ohio, 1993. 90% were vaccinated. Only 10% were not.
Source: N.Z. Miller; *"Vaccine Safety Manual"*; N.A. Press; Sante Fe, NM; pp. 140 (2008) (Refers to CDC and Official Surveillance data)

- Mumps outbreak in New York and New Jersey, 2010. 77% vaccinated. Only 23% were not. Source: *CNN news report*, Leslie Terjesen - Ocean county, NJ spokeswoman

- Measles, Ghana, 1972. 96% vaccinated. Only 4% were not. In 1967 the *World Health Organization* declared Ghana to be "measles free" due to the 96% vaccination rate, yet in 1972 one of the worst measles outbreaks in its history happened, killing more people than ever before.

- The November 1990 issue of *"Journal of the American Medical Association"* states: "Although more than 95% of school-age children in the US are vaccinated against measles, large measles outbreaks continue to occur in schools, and most cases in this setting occur among previously vaccinated children."

- "In 2006 an outbreak of mumps occurred in the US and amazingly the majority of cases were individuals that had received two vaccine doses." **Source**: "Human Vaccines; Volume 5; Issue 7 (2009); "Mumps outbreaks in highly vaccinated populations: What makes good even better?" pp. 494-496

- "A groundbreaking study published in the journal '*Clinical Infectious Diseases*', whose authorship includes scientists working for the Bureau of Immunization, New York City Department of Health and Mental Hygiene, and the National Center for Immunization and Respiratory Diseases, Centers for Disease Control and Prevention (CDC), Atlanta, GA, looked at evidence from the 2011 New York measles outbreak that individuals with prior evidence of measles vaccination and vaccine immunity were both capable of being infected with measles and infecting others with it (secondary transmission)." **Source**: *http://www.greenmedinfo.com/blog/measles-transmitted-vaccinated-gov-researchers-confirm*

I'd love to keep droning on and on and on and on like the energizer bunny, but that would just be a waste of my time. Examples like this are seemingly never ending! To make my point clear I will simply ask you to do a *Google.com* search for "disease outbreaks in highly vaccinated populations" and then take a look at the links provided. Go ahead, I'll wait...

When I did the search it yielded 29,500,000 results making it *very clear* that disease outbreaks *far too commonly* occur among the vaccinated, as a matter of fact it seems that they happen among the vaccinated more than anywhere else (just an honest, unbiased observation!).

Even Jonas Salk, *inventor of the polio vaccine*, testified before a Senate subcommittee that nearly all polio outbreaks since 1961 were *caused by the oral polio vaccine*. In 1985, the CDC (*Centers for Disease Control and Prevention*) reported that 87% of the cases of polio in the U.S. between 1973 and 1983 were *caused by the vaccine*, and later declared that all but a few imported cases since were caused by the vaccine, and most of the imported cases *occurred in fully immunized individuals*. I'm not making this stuff up, these are government sources.

Up until 1853 in England there were only regional outbreaks of smallpox, nothing close to an epidemic. But after smallpox vaccination was made mandatory in 1853 massive epidemics started happening. Between 1857 and 1859 there were over 14,000 deaths from smallpox. Between 1863 and 1865 there were over 20,000 smallpox deaths. Between 1870 and 1872 there were over 45,000 smallpox deaths. Official estimates as presented by Ann Riley Hale in her book *The Medical Voodoo* are that over

97% of the British population had been vaccinated, and official government documents indicate that the more people got vaccinated, the more they died from smallpox. The vaccine was made mandatory in Japan in 1872, twenty years later there were more than 165,000 cases of smallpox including over 30,000 deaths. In contrast, when Australia banned the vaccine in the 1800's cases of smallpox became nearly *unheard of*. No vaccine, no smallpox. Gee, what a coincidence!

An article from *NaturalNews.com* entitled *"Survey: Vaccinated children five times more prone to disease than unvaccinated children"* states the following:

> "An ongoing study out of Germany comparing disease rates among vaccinated and unvaccinated children points to a pretty clear disparity between the two groups as far as illness rates are concerned. As reported by the group Health Freedom Alliance, children who have been vaccinated according to official government schedules are up to five times more likely to contract a preventable disease than children who developed their own immune systems naturally without vaccines."

> **Full article is here**:*http://www.naturalnews.com/038647_vaccinated_children_disease _risk_unvaccinated.html#ixzz2Wi4IZ7U2*

Additionally, I'd like to point out that in the industrialized world the USA has the *highest vaccination rate* but has the *highest mortality (death) rate* for children under the age of 5. Sweden and Japan have the *lowest vaccination rates* and the *lowest mortality rates*. The champion of *infant* (first year of life) mortality rates is the USA as well. A recent article from *WashingtonPost.com* states:

> "The United States has a higher infant mortality rate than any of the other 27 wealthy countries, according to a new report from the Centers for Disease Control. A baby born in the U.S. is nearly three times as likely to die during her first year of life as one born in Finland or Japan. That same American baby is about twice as likely to die in her first year as a Spanish or Korean one.

> Despite healthcare spending levels that are significantly higher than any other country in the world, a baby born in the U.S. is less likely to see his first birthday than one born in Hungary, Poland or Slovakia. Or in Belarus. Or in Cuba, for that matter.

> The U.S. rate of 6.1 infant deaths per 1,000 live births masks considerable state-level variation. If Alabama were a country, its rate of 8.7 infant deaths per 1,000 would place it slightly behind Lebanon in the world rankings. Mississippi, with its 9.6 deaths, would be somewhere between Botswana and Bahrain.

> We're the wealthiest nation in the world. How did we end up like this?"

> **Full article is here**: *http://www.washingtonpost.com/blogs/wonkblog/wp/2014/09/29/ our-infant-mortality-rate-is-a-national-embarrassment/*

And last, but not least, from the mainstream media at *CBSNews.com* we have the following:

"A new report reveals that the United States has the highest first-day infant death rate out of all the industrialized countries in the world. About 11,300 newborns die within 24 hours of their birth in the U.S. each year, 50 percent more first-day deaths than all other industrialized countries combined, the report's authors stated."

Full article is here: *http://www.cbsnews.com/news/us-has-highest-first-day-infant-mortality-out-of-industrialized-world-group-reports/*

USA is # 1! **Numero uno** in *first day* deaths, *first year* deaths and *first 5 year* deaths. For a country that supposedly has the "greatest healthcare system in the world" I think I see a problem, don't you? If you don't you're not thinking clearly. If you don't see a problem yet then you have a *bias*, and *biases serve no purpose*.

You might be thinking that what I've presented so far is "only correlation science". You might think that I'm unfairly cherry picking data. You might be thinking "there's no proof that vaccines caused those deaths" yada yada yada. But I do find it interesting that the largest outbreaks of disease occur among the vaccinated, don't you? *The country that gives the most vaccines has the most deaths*. Hmmm. Very interesting indeed. Vaccines are supposed to *prevent disease*, but it does indeed seem to have the *direct opposite* effect. Again, thousands of examples can be cited. If vaccines work so well, if they're such a marvel of modern science, then why is it possible to come up with a seemingly never ending list of examples demonstrating the *utter failure of vaccines*? Call me crazy, but I just don't think that it should be that way. I think that if vaccines work then such failures shouldn't be so heavily documented. It just shouldn't be so easy to do a quick Google search and come up with *thousands of examples of vaccine failure* in about 5 seconds. Something is clearly *wrong* here!

"If we check back in history to that 1918 flu period (the great flu pandemic of 1918), we will see that it suddenly struck just after the end of World War I when our soldiers were returning home from overseas. That was the first war in which all the known vaccines were forced on all the servicemen. This mish-mash of poison drugs and putrid protein of which the vaccines were composed, caused such widespread disease and death among the soldiers that it was the common talk of the day, that more of our men were being killed by medical shots than by enemy shots from guns. Thousands were invalided home or to military hospitals, as hopeless wrecks, before they ever saw a day of battle. The death and disease rate among the vaccinated soldiers was four times higher than among the unvaccinated civilians. But this did not stop the vaccine promoters. Vaccine has always been big business, and so it was continued doggedly.

It was a shorter war than the vaccine-makers had planned on, only about a year for us, so the vaccine promoters had a lot of unused, spoiling vaccines left over which they wanted to sell at a good profit. So they did what they usually do, they called a meeting behind closed doors, and plotted the whole sordid program, a nationwide (worldwide) vaccination drive using all their vaccines, and telling the people that the soldiers were coming home with many dreaded diseases contracted in foreign countries and that it was the patriotic duty of every man, woman and child to get 'protected' by rushing down to the vaccination centers and having all the shots.

Most people believe their doctors and government officials, and do what they say. The result was, that almost the entire population submitted to the shots without question, and it was only a matter of hours until people began dropping dead in agony, while many others collapsed with a disease of such virulence that no one had ever seen anything like it before. They had all the characteristics of the diseases they had been vaccinated against, the high fever, chills, pain, cramps, diarrhea, etc. of typhoid, and the pneumonia like lung and throat congestion of diphtheria and the vomiting, headache, weakness and misery of hepatitis from the jungle fever shots, and the outbreak of sores on the skin from the smallpox shots, along with paralysis from all the shots, etc."

Source: *Vaccination the Silent Killer: A Clear and Present Danger* 1977, by Ida Honorof and E. McBean, page 28

The chart below not only shows the great pandemic caused by the forced vaccination of soldiers during WWI and the mass vaccinations that followed, it also clearly shows that vaccines had absolutely nothing to do with the decline of any diseases.

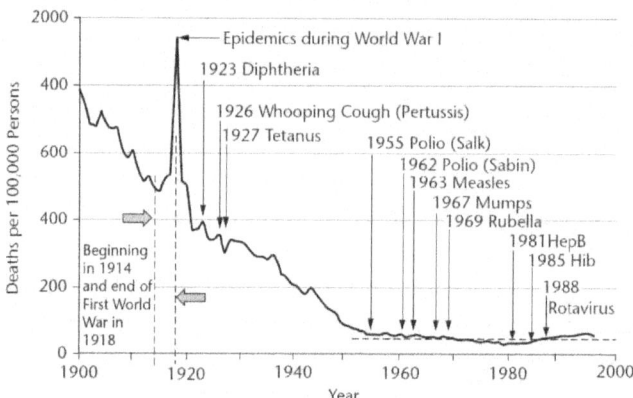

"Medical history books, almost uniformly extol the virtues of vaccination. Upon reading these books, one is left with the impression that during the 1800s and into the 1900s, there were rampant plagues that killed countless scores of people and that, because of vaccines, this is no longer the case. This is certainly what we believed growing up, and most people we talk to have a similar impression. It generally permeates society as an established fact."

- Suzanne Humphries, M.D.

If you have the belief that vaccines somehow "saved us" in the past, or that they work to prevent disease, you're mistaken. The data clearly shows that disease rates were *naturally* taking a nose dive long before the vaccines were introduced (see graph above).

This was due to improved sanitation among other things. As technology improved, so did human health, which only makes sense. A fine example of high disease rates due to poor sanitation in the modern world would be Africa. Their lack of clean water and modern sanitation technology has much to do with their disease rates, which are among the highest in the world. In the early 1900's sanitation technology wasn't nearly as efficient, it was on about the same level as Africa (ok maybe a little better depending on what part of Africa we're talking about), hence the higher disease rates, but as technology improved and better sanitation became the norm, disease rates naturally declined. Vaccines had *nothing* to do with it! As was clearly illustrated above, vaccines *promote* illness, they *do not* prevent anything!

Based upon what I've presented so far, it's not looking too good for vaccines, and I haven't even gotten to the good stuff yet. My ammo bag is still quite full.

They call them "immunizations" but where is the evidence that they cause people to become "immune" to disease? Again, the *direct opposite seems to be the case*, based upon the indisputable facts that you can see with a simple 5 second Google search. If they really do promote "immunity", as advertised, then why all of the outbreaks in highly vaccinated populations? Why are there *thousands* of interesting "coincidences" where people who get vaccinated *get the very disease they're vaccinated against*? And why would anyone want to dispute or deny that, much less insist upon getting vaccines for themselves or their children? That's sheer insanity! Don't get mad at me, I'm simply pointing out the truth. Is your ego and your need to be right about this issue more important than your own health and the health of your children? I certainly hope not. I certainly hope that you can read this with an open mind and learn the truth so that you can *protect* yourself and your children! Vaccines are a fraud. They promote disease. Accept it. It's true. They also make drug companies billions and billions and billions in profits! If you've read this book straight through from the beginning, I think you'll notice that a bit of a pattern is emerging concerning drug companies and profit margins, yes?

As for the infant mortality rates mentioned above, let's review the ingredients most commonly found in vaccines. This is straight from *CDC.gov*:

"Common substances found in vaccines include:

- **Aluminum**: gels or salts of aluminum which are added as adjuvants to help the vaccine stimulate a better response. Adjuvants help promote an earlier, more potent response, and more persistent immune response to the vaccine.

- **Antibiotics**: which are added to some vaccines to prevent the growth of germs (bacteria) during production and storage of the vaccine. No vaccine produced in the United States contains penicillin.

- **Egg protein**: is found in influenza and yellow fever vaccines, which are prepared using chicken eggs. Ordinarily, persons who are able to eat eggs or egg products safely can receive these vaccines.

- **Formaldehyde**: is used to inactivate bacterial products for toxoid vaccines, (these are vaccines that use an inactive bacterial toxin to produce immunity.) It is also used to kill unwanted viruses and bacteria that might contaminate the vaccine during production.

- **Monosodium glutamate (MSG) and 2-phenoxy-ethanol**: which are used as stabilizers in a few vaccines to help the vaccine remain unchanged when the vaccine is exposed to heat, light, acidity, or humidity.

- **Thimerosal**: is a mercury-containing preservative that is added to vials of vaccine that contain more than one dose to prevent contamination and growth of potentially harmful bacteria.

For children with a prior history of allergic reactions to any of these substances in vaccines, parents should consult their child's healthcare provider before vaccination."

Full article is here: _http://www.cdc.gov/vaccines/vac-gen/additives.htm_

There is no safe dosage level for _formaldehyde_, it can cause _leukemia and other cancers_, as well as _nervous system damage, brain damage, blindness and seizures. MSG is a brain toxin that attacks neurons._ You've already seen what I had to say about _antibiotics_ (in the MRSA section) and putting _aluminum_ in the blood stream is one of the worst things that you can do to a human being. _Aluminum_ poisoning causes the _loss of intellectual function; forgetfulness, memory loss, inability to concentrate, and in extreme cases, full blown dementia._ And isn't it interesting that many of the symptoms related to most of the above vaccine ingredients correlate with and are almost identical to the symptoms of _autism_?

"Did you know that the FDA Safety Level for Aluminum Exposure on a brand new child is 20 micrograms? That's the FDA safety level, meaning anything over 20 micrograms can cause severe neurological injury for an infant. Did you know that the shot given in the hospital before a baby is released, the Hepatitis B vaccine, contains 225 micrograms of aluminum? I bet you didn't know that. And you know what the problem is? Most parents don't know that."

- Mary Tocco, Vaccine expert for over 30 years, owner and operator of _ChildhoodShots.com_

They usually give that shot to babies on the _first day_ of life!

Never mind that it contains *11 times the limit set by the FDA* for safety, and never mind that the child's **blood-brain barrier** isn't working yet! Now go back and look at the symptoms of aluminum poisoning again. Go ahead, I'll wait...

As if aluminum isn't enough to worry about, we also have *mercury*, one of the most toxic and poisonous substances known to humankind as an ingredient in a shot that they give to infants! Did you know that there are 25 mcg of mercury included in almost every vaccine while the EPA sets the toxicity limit of mercury at .1 mcg? I'll do the math for you; almost every vaccine contains *__250 times__* *the toxicity limit of mercury* set by the EPA. As far as the so-called "mercury free" ones are concerned the FDA made a new rule stating that the vaccine manufacturers don't have to list it as an ingredient on the label unless it's used as a preservative! Most vaccines do, in fact, still contain, at the *bare minimum*, "trace" amounts of mercury.

The symptoms of mercury poisoning include:

- Loss of speech
- Social withdrawl
- Reduced eye contact
- Repetitive behaviors
- Hand-flapping, Toe walking
- Temper tantrums
- Sleep disturbances
- Seizures

The symptoms of autism include:

- Loss of speech
- Social withdrawl
- Reduced eye contact
- Repetitive behaviors
- Hand-flapping, Toe walking
- Temper tantrums
- Sleep disturbances
- Seizures

You might want to go back and look at those lists again. What did you notice? Yes, they're both *identical* to each other.

Despite the claims of "removing mercury" from vaccines in the early 2000's, cases of autism have only been skyrocketing. In 1983, according to the CDC's official vaccine schedule, there were a total of only 10 vaccines given to children under the age of 6 and the autism rate was only *__1 in 10,000__*. As of 2008 there were 36 vaccines given to children under the age of 6 and the autism rate had gone up to *1 in 150*. As of March 28th, 2014 there are 49 vaccines given to children under the age of 6 and we see the following:

> "*One in 68* U.S. children has an autism spectrum disorder (ASD), a 30% increase from 1 in 88 two years ago, according to a new report released Thursday by the Centers for Disease Control and Prevention."
>
> Full article here: *http://www.cnn.com/2014/03/27/health/cdc-autism/*

So the USA is not only # 1 in killing children (see above), it's # *1 in giving them autism* with bullshit vaccines. Autism is an epidemic in this country. I personally have two children in my family that are autistic, my sister's boy and one of my cousin's boys. It seems everyone knows someone who has an autistic child these days. We can't just ignore the ingredients in vaccines and the correlations between higher numbers of vaccines and higher rates of autism. Allow me to point out the fact that most of the ingredients that I mentioned above are toxic to brain function. Go back and read it one more time! And even if mercury really was "removed" from the vaccines, the *other* ingredients still remain! They include:

> **2-Phenoxyethanol**: A carcinogen, a developmental and reproductive toxicant. A metabolic poison, it interferes with the metabolism of all cells, the primary factor in the formation of cancer cells. It is capable of disabling the immune system's primary response.
>
> **Ammonium Sulfate**: A carcinogen. Ammonium sulfate is prepared by mixing ammonia with sulfuric acid. It is used as a chemical fertilizer for alkaline soils to lower the pH. In the body, it stresses the immune system by causing acidosis. Ammonium sulfate is also a liver toxicant, neurotoxicant, and respiratory toxicant.
>
> **Amphotericin B**: Can cause irreversible kidney damage, and mild liver failure. It has been known to produce severe histamine (allergic) reactions. There are several reports of anemia and cardiac failure. It is used used to treat fungus infections. Other side effects include blood clots, blood defects, kidney problems, nausea and fever. When used on the skin, allergic reactions can occur.
>
> **Animal Organ Tissue and Animal Blood**: Animal cells are used to culture the viruses in vaccines, so animal tissues and impurities are included in the formulation that is injected. Injections contain many types of animal viruses including monkey (kidney), cow (heart), calf (serum), chicken (embryo and egg), duck (egg), pig (blood), sheep (blood), dog (kidney), horse (blood), rabbit (brain), and guinea pig.
>
> **Animal Viruses**: The most documented is the monkey virus SV40. The virus is harmless in monkeys, but it stimulates rare cancers when injected into humans; brain cancer, bone (multiple myeloma), lungs (mesothelioma), and lymphoid tissue (lymphoma).

Antifreeze (ethylene glycol): Like what you put in your car! Classified as a "very toxic material".

Aspartame (Artificial Sweetener): Converts to formaldehyde in the body. Associated with numerous side effects including headache, dizziness, nausea, abdominal pain, blurred vision, memory loss, fatigue, hives, itching, numbness, breathing difficulty and seizures. For more details on aspartame see *Appendix C.*

Beta-Propiolactone: A carcinogen, a gastrointestinal and liver toxicant, respiratory toxicant, skin toxicant, and sense organ toxicant. More hazardous than most chemicals earning a 3 out of 3 in ranking systems. It appears on at least 5 federal regulatory lists. It is ranked as one of the most hazardous compounds to humans.

Borax (sodium tetraborate decahydrate): Traditionally used as a pesticide, it is a cardiovascular or blood toxicant, endocrine toxicant, gastrointestinal toxicant, liver toxicant and neurological toxicant. It was found to cause reproductive damage and reduced fertility in rats. It is banned in foods in the United States due to its toxicity. It is toxic to all cells, and has a slow excretion rate through the kidneys.

Foreign DNA: DNA from animals, viruses, fungi, and bacteria. Again, this is hazardous to the human body and alters DNA!

Genetically Modified Yeast: Genetically modified *anything* is hazardous to the human body and alters DNA!

Glutaraldehyde: Toxic, causing severe eye, nose, throat and lung irritations, along with headaches, drowsiness, and dizziness. The effects mirror the chemical warfare agent known as nerve gas. It is poisonous if ingested, and known to cause birth defects in experimental animals.

Large Foreign Proteins: In addition to the animal tissue impurities, there are large proteins that are deliberately included and used as adjuvants. Egg albumin and gelatin are in several vaccines. Casein (a milk protein) is in the triple antigen (DPT) vaccine. When injected, these normally harmless proteins are toxic to the body.

Latex: Latex in vaccines triggers allergic reactions to common products, like baby pacifiers, and is associated with the rise in those kind of allergies.

Live Human Viruses: Live viruses in vaccines are sometimes claimed to be killed, inactivated, or attenuated. Not true. The method used to inactivate viruses is treatment with formaldehyde. Its effectiveness is temporary. Once injected into the body, the formaldehyde is broken down, releasing the virus in its original state. It is documented in orthodox medical literature that the "crippled" viruses can revert to their former virulence, which explains why vaccines cause the very diseases they are said to "prevent".

Methanol: A volatile, flammable, poisonous liquid alcohol. It is used as a solvent in industry, and as an antifreeze compound in fuel. In the body it is metabolized into formaldehyde.

Mycoplasma: Microscopic organisms are considered to be the smallest free-moving organisms. Many are pathogenic, and one species is the cause of mycoplasma pneumonia which is noted to occur "only in children and young adults" according to Mosby's Medical Dictionary.

Phenol: A carcinogen, and a cardiovascular and blood toxicant. A developmental toxin, gastrointestinal toxin, liver toxin, kidney toxin, neurotoxin, respiratory toxin, skin and sense organ toxin. It has been placed on at least 8 federal regulatory watch lists.

<u>**Polysorbate 20/80 Emulsifier**</u>: A known skin and sense organ toxin. Verified as a cancer causing agent in animals.

<u>**Sorbitol (Artifical Sweetener)**</u>: Diabetic retinopathy and neuropathy may be related to excess sorbitol in the cells of the eyes and nerves, leading to blindness. This is another suspected carcinogen. Sorbitol is a gastrointestinal and liver toxicant.

<u>**Sulfate and Phosphate Compounds**</u>: Can trigger severe allergies in children, which may last throughout their lives to permanently impair their immune systems.

<u>**Tri(n)butylphosphate**</u>: A carcinogen, a kidney toxicant and a neurotoxicant. It is more hazardous than most chemicals in 2 out of 3 ranking systems. It is on at least 1 federal regulatory list.

If you can look at this list of ingredients and not be alarmed then there's clearly something wrong with *your* brain function! Perhaps you've had a few too many vaccines yourself? Granted, there are other factors, other things that can cause autism that have changed over the years such as GMO and chemical laden "foods", fluoride and chlorine in drinking water, etc. but by far the biggest factor that has changed since 1983 is the *number of vaccines* given to the kids! Based upon the long list of *neurotoxins and brain damage inducing substances that they contain* I really don't think it's much of a stretch to say that vaccines are causing the rise in autism. I really don't believe that fact should be considered "controversial"! I do believe it's as obvious as the sky being blue that vaccines cause autism. As a matter of fact, on the package insert of the *Sanoi Pasteur DTaP* vaccine (Diphtheria, Tetanus and Pertussis) dated from Dec. 2005 says the following:

> "Adverse events reported during post-approval use of Tripedia vaccine include idiopathic thrombocytopenic, purpura, **SIDS (sudden infant death symdrome!), anaphylactic reaction (a severe, life threatening allergic reaction!)**, cellulitis, **autism, convulsion/grand mal convulsion**, encephalopathy, hypotonia, neuropathy, somnolence and apnea. Events were included in this list because of the **seriousness or frequency of reporting**."

Emphasis was mine. Remember, this isn't me, this is an **actual package insert on a vaccine** openly admitting that it causes SIDS, autism, life threatening allergic reactions, grand mal seizures and more! And then it says that they put those warnings on there because of the *frequency* and *seriousness* of the reports that they've received!

The list of ingredients on the insert says:

"Diphtheria and Tetanus Toxoids and Acellular Pertussis Vaccine Absorbed
Tripedia, Sanofi Pasteur, Inc., Dec. 2005: sodium phosphate, peptone-based medium,
bovine extract (US sourced), **formaldehyde**, ammonium sulfate, aluminum potassium
sulfate, modified Mueller and Miller medium, modified Stainer-Scholte medium, isotonic
sodium, chloride solution, sodium phosphate, **thimerosal (trace)**, gelatin, polysorbate 80
(Tween 80), **aluminum**"

Take note that they also admit to "trace" amounts of mercury
(thimerosal), despite the claim that mercury was "removed" from
vaccines in the early 2000's, and even the FDA admits that
mercury is still used in vaccines on its website:

"While the use of mercury-containing preservatives has declined in recent years with the
development of new products formulated with alternative or no preservatives, thimerosal
has been used in some immune globulin preparations, anti-venins, skin test antigens, and
ophthalmic and nasal products, in addition to **certain vaccines**."

Full article is here: *http://www.fda.gov/BiologicsBloodVaccines/SafetyAvailability/
VaccineSafety/UCM096228#thi*

A recent study from April of 2012 clearly demonstrated that
*"Baby Monkeys Develop Autism Symptoms After Getting Popular
Childhood Vaccines"*:

"Following a recent study conducted by scientists at the University of Pittsburgh,
Pennsylvania which revealed that many infant monkeys given standard doses of
childhood vaccines as part of the new research, developed autism symptoms, question
marks over the ultimate safety of vaccines have come to the fore.

The groundbreaking research findings presented at the International Meeting for Autism
Research (IMFAR) in London, England, have revealed that young macaque monkeys
given the typical CDC-recommended vaccination schedule from the 1990s, and in
appropriate doses for the monkeys' sizes and ages, tended to develop autism symptoms.
Their unvaccinated counterparts, on the other hand, developed no such symptoms, which
points to a strong connection between vaccines and autism spectrum disorders."

Full article is here: *http://www.fhfn.org/baby-monkeys-develop-autism-symptoms-after-
getting-popular-childhood-vaccines/*

There is simply too much evidence against vaccines to try and
defend them folks! Let's move on to adult shots. Did you get your
flu shot this year? Here's another package insert for you. This one
is from the *FLULAVAL* (Influenza Virus Vaccine) 2011-2012
formula:

"...there have been **no controlled trials** adequately demonstrating a decrease in influenza
disease after vaccination with FLULAVAL."

So here we have a vaccine manufacturer admitting that there is *no
science* behind the vaccine. *None!* "No controlled trials". Is that
clear enough for you? And I really hate to tell you the truth (wait,
no I don't!) but there are no scientific studies or random controlled

trials available for any vaccine, period. *None.* There are, of course, Big Pharma "studies" that were funded by Big Pharma *themselves,* with cooked, fraudulent and cherry picked data that they use as "proof" for the efficacy of *their own products*! I've already shown you (in the book's introduction) the amount of fraud that is involved in the medical journals and in their safety reports. Talk about a *huge* conflict of interest! If you believe in vaccines even after reading what I've said so far, I challenge you to find me an *independent* study from an *unbiased* source and email it to me: kenny@loveevolvetranscend.com. I'm looking for ***any independent, unbiased study*** that proves the safety and efficacy of ***any vaccine***. Send it to me, if you can find one! Have fun looking because you won't find one!

And because of the fact that there are no studies to prove the safety and efficacy of vaccines, believing in them requires *faith*, and it requires *faith* because there is *no science* to rely on! *Faith* in "doctors", *faith* in the government's "advice" and *faith* in vaccine manufacturers. It's the *Church of Medicinal Quackery* and vaccine *believers* are their flock of *sheep*. I personally don't believe in taking things on faith, especially when it involves pumping neurotoxins like mercury, aluminum, antifreeze and formaldehyde into my body and the bodies of innocent children! I've presented enough evidence so far in this book to convince anyone with any intelligence whatsoever that vaccines simply are not what they are claimed to be; they are *dangerous*, they are *not effective,* they *promote disease,* they *promote autism,* they *kill and maim innocent people,* and they shouldn't be used under any circumstances. *Ever!* If you're still skeptical then you're clearly brainwashed. If you still believe in vaccines after what I've said about them here then there's no hope for you whatsoever. You can believe whatever you want, but I pity your children, *especially if they end up a statistic because of you.*

A study published in the Oct. 2008 issue of *Archives of Pediatric and Adolescent Medicine* concluded that:

"significant influenza vaccine effectiveness could not be demonstrated for any season, age or setting".

Another study in the Sept. 2008 issue of *American Journal of Respiratory and Critical Care Medicine* confirmed that there has been *no decrease in deaths* from influenza and pneumonia in the elderly regardless of the fact that vaccination rates have risen from 15% in 1980 to 65% in 2008.

A large scale, systematic review of 51 studies involving over 260,000 children was published in the *Cochrane Database of Systematic Reviews* in 2006. They found that there is *zero evidence* that the flu vaccine is any more effective than a placebo in children aged 6 months to 2 years. In other words, *zero percent effective*! So why risk injecting mercury, aluminum, antifreeze and formaldehyde into your child for no benefit?

The same people also reviewed 64 studies covering a 40 year period and reported that for elderly people living in nursing homes, flu shots provided *"little or no effectiveness"* at preventing the flu!

Let's recap this section; first I demonstrated that huge outbreaks of disease regularly happen in highly vaccinated populations. Then I demonstrated that the USA, being the highest vaccinated population in the world, also has the highest percentage of death rates in the industrialized world for children on **1)** their first day **2)** their first year and **3)** their first 5 years. I showed you the list of *toxic shit* contained in vaccines, in particular mercury and aluminum, and how far over the "safety limits" they are, even by the government's own standards. I showed undeniable correlations between increased vaccination rates and increased rates of autism, and I even showed you that at least one vaccine manufacturer openly admits that their vaccine causes SIDS, autism, severe allergic reactions, and grand mal seizures. I also showed you that there is no science behind vaccines, nor is there any evidence that they actually prevent illness. I showed you that the opposite is true, that they cause illness, injuries, autism and death. Not so good for a "miracle of modern science" huh? So why do they allow this to continue? I know that his might be getting old, if you've been reading this book from page one, but have you been following the money trail?

"The Alliance Between the Vaccine Industry and the Government

In the first quarter of 2010 alone, the US federal government representatives received $19 million per day from lobbyists, and over $1 billion in total lobbyist spending, a large chunk of the money coming from the health care sector.

Keep in mind, this is only federal lobbying efforts. This figure doesn't take into account the millions more spent lobbying at the state level, not to mention the cozy lobbying arrangements between the drug reps and individual doctors.

Why this massive lobbying push by the vaccine industry?

One of the reasons (certainly not the only one), is to influence vaccine mandates. The vaccine industry has a vested interest in (and continually spends big money on) trying to make sure that more vaccines and more doses are mandated by the government.

For every mandate they have successfully pushed through, there are some recent ones that have failed due to action taken by parents of vaccine injured children and others to defeat them.

Currently in California, there is a bill under consideration to make pertussis vaccine booster doses mandatory for all children between 7th and 12th grade.

And in New York there has been a battle over a bill to make flu shots mandatory for all health care workers, and those who refuse an annual flu shot stand to lose their job.

There are also a whopping 145 additional vaccines in the pipeline being developed and tested in clinical trials. Since drug companies are going to want a stable, predictable market in the U.S. for these new vaccines, they're likely to press for mandated use of many of them, both by children and adults."

Full article is here: *http://articles.mercola.com/sites/articles/archive/2010/11/04/big-profits-linked-to-vaccine-mandates.aspx*

The vaccine industry brought in ***25 billion dollars*** in profits in 2013, and they're predicted to be up to ***48 billion*** by 2017. What have I been saying about drug company profits in this book? And remember, the people who own the drug companies also own the mainstream press, and the "educational" institutions that train the "doctors", etc. and you also saw that they buy off our politicians spending millions per day to get what they want. Can you say "corrupt" everybody? Can you say "crime against humanity" everybody? And low and behold, just take a look at what we have here! Talk about a *glaring* conflict of interest! A brand new article entitled *"Former CDC Director Julie Gerberding sells 38,368 shares of Merck Stock for $2.3 Million"* from May 25th, 2015:

"Julie Gerberding was in charge of the Centers for Disease Control and Prevention (CDC) from 2002 to 2009, which includes the years the FDA approved the Merck Gardasil vaccine. Soon after she took over the CDC, she reportedly completely overhauled the agency's organizational structure, and many of the CDC's senior scientists and leaders either left or announced plans to leave. Some have claimed that almost all of the replacements Julie Gerberding appointed had ties to the vaccine industry.

Gerberding resigned from the CDC on January 20, 2009, and took over as the president of Merck's Vaccine division, a 5 billion dollar a year operation, and the supplier of the largest number of vaccines the CDC recommends (Article here: *http://www.xconomy.com/national/2011/06/24/mercks-julie-gerberding-former-cdc-director-on-the-future-of-vaccines/*).

It was reported earlier this month (May 11th, 2015) that Dr. Gerberding, now the executive vice president of pharmaceutical giant Merck, sold 38,368 of her shares in Merck stock for $2,340,064.32. She still holds 31,985 shares of the company's stock, valued at about $2 million. (**Source**: *http://www.dakotafinancialnews.com/merck-co-evp-julie-l-gerberding-sells-38368-shares-mrk/159207/*)

Besides examples like this showing a clear conflict of interest between government agencies tasked with overseeing public health and vaccine safety and pharmaceutical companies, the National Institute of Health also holds patents on vaccines such as Gardasil, and earns royalties from the sale of vaccines."

Full article is here: *http://vaccineimpact.com/2015/former-cdc-director-julie-gerberding-sells-38368-shares-of-merck-stock-for-2-3-million/*

Clearly, this should be illegal. This is as criminal as it gets. She rigged the game for herself as director of the CDC, invested in vaccines and loaded up her staff with people from the vaccine industry. After she left as director of the CDC she cashed in on it, and she still has financial ties to vaccine profits. If it was up to me she'd be **in prison for a long, long time**, but this country is so corrupt she's getting away with it and nobody has anything to say about it. It's *business as usual*.

Additionally, laws have been passed *releasing drug companies from all liability*. On Feb. 22, 2011 the *US Supreme Court* shielded Big Pharma from *all liability* for vaccine injuries and deaths! If you have a child who turns autistic or dies after being vaccinated, guess what? You're shit out of luck. If you become paralyzed after receiving a flu shot, which is all too common believe it or not, then guess what? You're shit out of luck. *No matter what happens* due to your choice to get vaccinated, you're shit out of luck. *You're on your own*!

If you have a child who is vaccine injured or "autistic" the best plan of action is an organic, low glycemic diet in combination with chelation therapy. The idea is to remove the toxic buildup from the system by cleansing and flushing the system. Chelation therapy binds to heavy metals and other toxins and flushes them. Intravenous EDTA chelation therapy is the fastest acting and the most potent, but it has a price tag of between two to five thousand dollars. Chances of getting it covered by insurance are slim, but it couldn't hurt to try. If you can't afford intravenous therapy there is also oral chelation therapy, which runs roughly $50.00 per month. Absorption and effectiveness of oral therapy is obviously much lower than intravenous, but if you take it on a regular basis for a long enough period, similar results can be achieved.

Another method of eliminating heavy metals from the system is chlorella and cilantro therapy. When both are used together it can be very effective for eliminating toxic buildup in the system. Cilantro serves to pull the toxins from the tissues and the chlorella acts as a binder and carrier of the toxins out of the system. Neither substance by itself would be of much benefit, but the two together are very powerful.

In closing; There is no credible scientific report or study that conclusively proves that vaccines prevent illness, there is only a bunch of propaganda and media hype with no science to back up the claims made. Nobody has scientifically proven the effectiveness of vaccines, ever. On the flip side, there are thousands of reports of people actually getting the very disease that they were vaccinated for *from the vaccine itself*. Children and adults alike are being permanently injured and/or dying from side effects of vaccines including paralysis, autism and sudden infant death syndrome (SIDS). At least four ingredients in vaccines are incredibly dangerous and 100% unfit for human consumption, mercury, aluminum, antifreeze and formaldehyde. There is *no safe dosage level* for *any* of those ingredients! It is ludicrous to even consider putting those substances into your body at any dosage! Now that I know what I know about vaccines I will *never* get a flu shot or vaccinate *ever again*! Even if I was shown scientific data and studies that vaccines really do *prevent* illness, which don't exist, I would continue to opt out of taking them in favor of natural and safe alternatives. If I ever have children they will be on daily doses of ***colloidal silver, antiviral and antibiotic herbs*** and other *safe* and *natural immune system boosters* for *real protection against disease!* I would allow their immune system to **develop naturally** instead of ***destroying it with toxic shit*** during the first years of their life when their bodies aren't even fully developed yet! As a responsible and intelligent human being I refuse to jeopardize the lives and health of myself and especially innocent children just for the sake of having *blind faith* in an unproven pseudoscience called vaccines! And neither should you! Wake up!

HIV Does Not Cause AIDS

"If there is evidence that HIV causes AIDS, there should be scientific documents which either singly or collectively demonstrate that fact, at least with a high probability. There is no such document."

- Dr. Kary Mullis, Biochemist, 1993 Nobel Prize for Chemistry

I am quite thoroughly convinced that the HIV=AIDS hypothesis is, like ADHD, an *invention* of Big Pharma. I believe that because of the scientific facts surrounding the issue. In 1984, the "cause" of AIDS was announced at a Press Conference by the Reagan White House, via Dr. Robert Gallo. Why did they bypass the scientific facts? No presentation, written paper or study has ever shown conclusively that HIV causes AIDS. Ever since then a group of censored scientists has questioned this hypothesis.

Dr. Kary Mullis is a *Nobel Prize-winning American biochemist*, author, and lecturer. In recognition of his invention of the polymerase chain reaction (PCR) technique he shared the 1993 *Nobel Prize in Chemistry* with Michael Smith and earned the Japan Prize in the same year. He very adamantly states that HIV absolutely does *not* cause AIDS.

"...I recognized that I did not know the scientific reference to support a statement I had just written: 'HIV is the probable cause of AIDS.' Of course, this simple reference had to be out there *somewhere*. There had to be a published paper, or perhaps several of them, which taken together indicated that HIV was the probable cause of AIDS. There just had to be. I did computer searches, but came up with nothing. I was going to a lot of meetings and conferences as part of my job. I got in the habit of approaching anyone who gave a talk about AIDS and asking him or her what reference I should quote for that increasingly problematic statement, 'HIV is the probable cause of AIDS.' After ten or fifteen meetings over a couple of years, I was getting pretty upset when *no one* could cite the reference. I didn't like the ugly conclusion that was forming in my mind: The entire campaign against a disease increasingly regarded as a twentieth-century Black Plague was based on a hypothesis whose origins no one could recall. That defied both scientific and common sense.

"Finally, I had the opportunity to question one of the giants in HIV and AIDS research, Dr. Luc Montagnier of the Pasteur Institute, when he gave a talk in San Diego. It would be the last time I would be able to ask my little question without showing anger, and I figured Montagnier would know the answer. So I asked him. With a look of condescending puzzlement, Montagnier said, 'Why don't you quote the report from the Centers for Disease Control?' I replied, 'It doesn't really address the issue of whether or not HIV is the probable cause of AIDS does it?' 'No,' he admitted, no doubt wondering when I would go away. He looked for support to the little circle of people around him, but they were all awaiting a more definitive response, like I was. 'Why don't you quote the work on SIV (Simian Immunodifficiency Virus)?' the good doctor offered. 'I read that too, Dr. Montagnier,' I responded. 'What happened to those monkeys didn't remind me of AIDS. Besides, that paper was just published only a couple of months ago. I'm looking for the *original paper* where somebody showed that HIV caused AIDS.' This time, Dr.

Montagnier's response was to walk quickly away to greet an aquaintance across the room."

- Quoted from the introduction to the book *Inventing the AIDS Virus* by Peter H. Duesberg

Peter H. Duesberg, Ph.D. is a professor of Molecular and Cell Biology at the *University of California*, Berkeley. He isolated the first cancer gene through his work on *retroviruses* (keep in mind that HIV is supposedly a *retrovirus!*) in 1970, and mapped the genetic structure of these viruses. Professor Duesberg partnered with Dr. Robert Gallo for cancer research, and they were friends for a long time. His cancer research got him elected to the *National Academy of Sciences* in 1986. He was also the recipient of a seven-year Outstanding Investigator Grant from the *National Institute of Health*. In 1987 he claimed that HIV is *not* the cause of AIDS.

"It was Dr. Peter Duesberg who first threw down the gauntlet in 1987 to challenge the huge and growing industry around the 'HIV causes AIDS' theory when he published a paper in the Journal of Cancer Research. He pointed out that; HIV does not destroy immune system T-cells in laboratory petri dishes, none of the 150 chimpanzees injected with HIV have AIDS, the growing number of HIV negative AIDS cases (now over 4,000 documented), only two percent of HIV positive hemophiliacs have AIDS symptoms, the same percentage as HIV negative hemophiliacs, that AZT (at that time the most expensive and only drug approved for HIV infections) was a known toxin with documented side effects which were attributed to AIDS, and that nearly every AIDS patient was known to be a frequent user of hard drugs."

- Stephen Simac

Professor Duesberg states that there is no scientific evidence for the HIV=AIDS hypothesis and says that HIV is in fact *biochemically inactive* rendering it *harmless*. He also points out that HIV is not behaving (spreading out into the population) as any contagious virus would. His scientific papers challenging the HIV=AIDS hypothesis have appeared in journals worldwide including *Journal of AIDS, AIDS Forschung, Biomedicine and Pharmacotherapeutics, Research in Immunology, Cancer Research, The New England Journal of Medicine, Science, Nature, The Lancet, British Medical Journal* and *Proceedings of the National Academy of Sciences*.

His conclusion is that AIDS is caused by long-term recreational drug use and/or HIV drugs themselves (*the "treatments"*) such as AZT, which destroy the immune system. The drug companies have refused to engage in scientific debate with Duesberg and the mainstream "scientific" community has pretty much ostracized him. For 23 years, before his first published paper questioning the HIV=AIDS hypothesis, he never had any funding requests turned down. Since that paper has come out he gets turned down for funding requests on a regular basis. And of course, his long time friend, Dr. Robert Gallo, has disowned him.

Pardon me but it seems that something fishy is going on here. Something here stinks. Dr. Kerry Mullis, the man who ***invented the PCR test*** searched for over two years for a simple report on why it is believed that HIV=AIDS, and he never found anything. When he questioned one of the top people in the field, Dr. Luc Montagnier, he was ignored. Professor Peter Duesberg has not only been ostracized from the scientific community, he has been refused every time he offers to discuss the science regarding HIV and AIDS. If there is adequate evidence that HIV causes AIDS then why would they refuse debate? If they have conclusive proof then why not jump all over the opportunity to present it to the public? If Professor Duesberg is wrong, if HIV really does cause AIDS and if the science proves it, then what are they afraid of? And why refuse his funding requests all of a sudden?

Dr. Mullis and Professor Duesberg are very prominent people in the world of science, every bit as prominent as Dr. Robert Gallo himself, and they have many good points regarding this issue. They have questions that have never been answered and they have facts that cannot be denied or ignored.

I personally have six reasons why I believe that HIV does *not* cause AIDS:

1) The *live* HIV virus has never been isolated from HIV/AIDS patients nor has it ever been photographed: HIV has never been isolated from the body of a human being. Period. Not the *active* virus, anyway. What has been done is this: They have found the *inactive* HIV "virus" in body tissue, *not in the blood*, and then used a long, drawn out, complicated chemical process to reactivate it. Take note of what Professor Duesberg said. He stated that HIV is an *inactive* virus and is harmless. It is! I have seen no evidence that he's mistaken, to the contrary he is 100% correct, because the *live virus* has never, *ever* been isolated!

"Up to today there is actually no single scientifically really convincing evidence for the existence of HIV. Not even once such a retrovirus has been isolated and purified by the methods of classical virology."

- Dr. Heinz Ludwig Sanger, Emeritus Professor of Molecular Biology and Virology, Max-Planck-Institutes for Biochemistry, Munchen

Question: If HIV is a "contagious virus" then why hasn't it been isolated from the blood of a patient? It should be a very simple procedure, if HIV is what they claim it to be, after all they can do that with *every other* contagious virus.

Also, they have never photographed HIV in the blood of a human being with an electron microscope. *Ever*! Don't you find that a bit disturbing?

"This embarrassing lack of electron microscope evidence for substantiating the nature of the so-called viral load in AIDS patients was first reported during an important AIDS conference that took place in Pretoria, S.A., in May 2000. None of the AIDS experts present at that conference could demonstrate the presence of retroviral particles in the blood of AIDS patients. Moreover, almost two years ago, a substantial award ($100,000) was officially offered to anybody who would demonstrate HIV particles in the blood of allegedly high viral load patients. Two years later, the award has still not been claimed."

- Henry Bauer, professor of chemistry and science studies at *Virginia Polytechnic Institute and State University*, 2003

2) The "tests" are about as accurate as a *coin toss* and the package inserts say that they are *"not intended to detect the presence of a virus"*. The "tests" have never been approved by the FDA as an accurate method to determine HIV infection. Numerous factors (too many to list) such as pregnancy, flu, malnutrition, hepatitis, MS, measles, pneumonia, antibiotic damage, Epstein Barr virus, glandular fever, malaria, syphilis, and over 50 other conditions can bring up false positive results.

"A diagnosis of 'HIV+' is like a diagnosis of 'Yes, he's breathing'".

- Liam Scheff, author of *Official Stories*

Coming up positive on an HIV "test" is simply not what most people believe it is, it has nothing to do with AIDS.

"So-called 'HIV tests' have not been proven to detect infection by HIV (human immunodeficiency virus, a retrovirus) even though for more than a quarter century these tests have been widely used to diagnose such infection. Manufacturers of the test kits do not claim that the tests detect infection. The tests are for and were approved only for screening blood, where sensitivity rather than specificity is the prime criterion and false positives are of relatively little concern. Technical discussion of how to detect HIV infection makes plain that in themselves the tests are insufficient to diagnose infection. In point of fact, 'positive HIV' tests may be the result of dozens of such conditions as hyper gamma, anemia, tuberculosis, vaccination against influenza, receipt of tetanus immune globulin, or even pregnancy."

Read full pdf file here: *www.cwbpi.com/AIDS/reports/HIVtestsBauer2010.pdf*

Read the fine print (on the "test" kit inserts):

ELISA Antibody Test insert: "At present there is no recognized standard for establishing the presence and absence of HIV-1 antibody in human blood." (No way to determine if HIV antibodies are in the blood? Huh?)

Western Blot "Confirmatory" Test insert: "Do not use this kit as the sole basis of diagnosing HIV-1 infection. Positive blot results using any specimen type should be followed with additional testing." (This is the "confirmatory" test? What the...)
The package insert on the Western Blot **also states**: "...in the general population, which the CDC estimates to have a prevalence of HIV infection of 0.006%, using a test with a specificity of 99%, the result is that **94% of all positives will be false positives**."

Amplicore HIV-1 Monitor: "...test is not intended to be used as a screening test for HIV or as a diagnostic test to confirm the presence of HIV infection." (This test is not intended to confirm the presence of the virus?)

PCR Genetic Test insert: "Not intended to be used as a screening test for HIV or as a diagnostic test to confirm the presence of HIV infection." (This test is not intended to confirm the presence of the virus?)

bDNA Genetic Test insert: "Not intended for use as a screening assay for HIV infection or as a diagnostic test to confirm the diagnosis of HIV infection." (This test is not intended to confirm the presence of the virus?)

Ok, so where is the real test then? The reason that the manufacturers put these disclaimers on their "tests" is simple; if someone tries to *sue* them all they would have to do is show them the package insert and flip them off. The tests are not designed to look for or find HIV, and the test inserts admit that in the fine print, but "doctors" still use them to tell people that they are "infected" with HIV and will soon get AIDS and die! Isn't that just fucking incredible? With something as critical as HIV/AIDS, don't you agree that they should test for the virus itself, or at the very least be certain that the virus is in the blood stream before they tell people that they are *going to die*?

I was tested once, and I remember being very, very afraid until I got the results. Back then I believed that HIV causes AIDS, and I was was very nervous until I found out that the test came back negative. If I would have been told I was HIV+ it would have devastated me! And that's what happens when people are "diagnosed" with HIV. They start dying right on the spot, quite literally, whether they have a disease or not, it's an incredibly emotional situation for them. Many people diagnosed as HIV+ *commit suicide*. Imagine being told that you have an incurable, deadly disease and that you're going to die. Just imagine that! And then take a look again at what it says on those test inserts, and try to convince me that that's ok! Oh yeah, no big deal! We can let that slide. Not! If it were *you*, would you trust the diagnosis, knowing what you now know about those "tests"?

As it is, they've never even pulled the live virus from the blood of a patient or even seen it under a microscope! How could this be a "contagious virus" if it can't be detected or proven to be in the blood of a patient? Once again, I'm calling it the way it is, this is a *crime against humanity*!

There have been numerous cases where people take an HIV test more than once, even several times, only to get differing results! First they're positive, and then they're negative, and then they're "inconclusive" and then they're positive again! In other cases people move from one state to another state and go from being HIV+ to being HIV- just because of a new geographic location! These "tests" are bullshit, they don't prove anything, and using them to tell people that they are going to die is a *ruthless* crime against the human race!

> "I don't recommend people ever get tested [for HIV]. The reason is, I don't know what the tests mean...no one else knows what the tests mean."
>
> - Robert Da Prato, MD, HIV Testing Specialist, US Army

3) As already mentioned above, there is not a single study to prove that HIV causes AIDS; not even from Dr. Robert Gallo, the "discoverer" that HIV causes AIDS. Dr. Luc Montagnier, Gallo's partner in the "HIV causes AIDS" theory, has since admitted in 1989:

> "We can be exposed to HIV many times without being chronically infected. Our immune system will get rid of the virus in a few weeks, if you have a good immune system." He also said: "*HIV is not capable of causing the destruction of the immune system* which is seen in people with AIDS."

Dr Robert E. Wilner, author of the book *The Deadly Deception: The Proof That Sex And HIV Absolutely Do Not Cause AIDS* even injected himself with HIV+ blood several times on television to support his claims and continued to test HIV- for many years after that until he eventually passed away from natural causes.

4) Diagnosing AIDS is purely unscientific based upon a list of characteristics that changes all the time and differs from country to country. You can have AIDS in the USA but if you go to Canada you will not because they have a different definition. They diagnose many people without even doing HIV tests right here in America. Many people who get diagnosed aren't even sick, they have a healthy immune system, etc. but then get diagnosed with full blown AIDS.

AIDS is not a virus, it is a syndrome! If you are HIV+ and you get pneumonia, they call it AIDS. If you are HIV- and you get pneumonia, they call it pneumonia. The same can be said for 28 other conditions that have existed long before the term "AIDS" was invented. The most basic definition of AIDS is that your immune system is compromised. This is nothing new. The only thing new about it is the term "AIDS". Millions of people have died in history from compromised immune systems, and many of them had the illnesses on the list of 29 AIDS illnesses as well, they just didn't call it "AIDS"!

In Africa people don't have much food or clean water, they don't have the most basic medicines, and they live in very unsanitary conditions. Of course people are going to get sick! Of course their immune systems will be compromised! They don't have anything they need! And then when they get sick the "doctors" don't even test their blood, they just say "Oh it must be AIDS." And there is your reason for the "AIDS epidemic" in Africa. It's not AIDS! It's the *same thing* that has been happening there for *hundreds of years* only they didn't call it AIDS! Give those people clean water, food and more sanitary conditions and then watch the "AIDS epidemic" as well as many other diseases go away! Remember what I said back in the vaccines section, as sanitation improves so does human health, it's a no brainer. It's not rocket science, it's called common sense.

5) The # 1 killer of HIV+ people is HIV "treatment" not AIDS! The toxic drugs they are given which *break down the immune system* are the number one killer! The drug AZT was invented as a cancer (chemotherapy) drug that proved to be so deadly toxic that the FDA wouldn't approve its use for human beings. It was later put through a bogus "trial" and even though *169 of the 172 trial participants* **died** they approved it *anyway* to give to HIV/AIDS patients. What a genius idea! Tell people they're dying from a disease that *destroys the immune system*, and then prescribe them with drugs that *destroy the immune system*! When they get sick and die just blame it on AIDS! And just look at how much money they make selling those drugs! The profits just keep rolling on in! What a great scam!

> "The most toxic drug that has ever been licensed for long term consumption in the free world. AZT is a prescription drug and according to the manufacturer itself it causes symptoms that are indistinguishable from AIDS. So I would say it is not arrogant for me to say that AZT is AIDS by prescription."
>
> - Professor Peter Duesberg

AZT was passed out like candy to tens of thousands of healthy people who were diagnosed HIV+ with those shady "tests" and then the AIDS death rate, *which had been declining* suddenly started going up again. Gee, I wonder why?

A journalist by the name of Celia Farber posed the following questions to a representative of *Glaxo*, the company that manufactures AZT:

> "I just want to know your perspective. If I were to say to you, that it seemed clear to us all in the late 80s, that people were dying very rapidly from high dose AZT – not from 'AIDS' but from high dose AZT, I mean 1200 mg, 1000 mg, and so forth, the early years...if I were to say that as a statement of fact, that high dose AZT was killing gay men outright in those years, would you think I was wrong?"

Are you ready for the drug rep's answer? Here it is:

> "Of course not. You'd be right. Why do you think we lowered the dose?"

After the dosage was officially lowered, the death rates from AIDS suddenly plunged back down to almost, but not quite, the same rates as before AZT was introduced. What an odd coincidence!

In July 2002 researchers at the *14th World AIDS Conference* revealed that the leading cause of death among HIV+ Americans was AZT:

> "Ninety-four percent of all AIDS-related deaths in the US occurred after the introduction of AZT," according to CDC statistics through the year 2000.

Here is an actual AZT label:

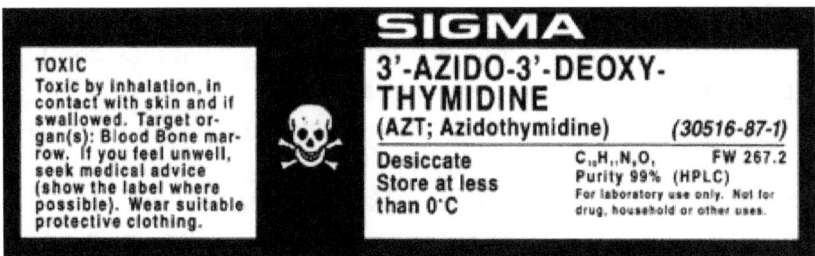

Nice "medicine" huh? Yeah, this will make you healthy! This is good for you! It's ok, you can trust me, I'm a "doctor"!

After they lowered the dosage for AZT they added the new "protease inhibitors". At the same *14th World AIDS Conference* in July 2002 researchers revealed:

> "According to the University of Pittsburgh, the number one cause of death in US AIDS patients today (2003) is liver failure, a side-effect of the new protease inhibitors."

Liam Scheff had this to say about it:

> "In the mid-90s, they added protease drugs, which alter physiology, melt the fat from the arms and face, leaving skin and bones, whittling muscle to nothing, redistributing fat into humps on the neck and back, bloating the stomach beyond proportion and making legs into toothpicks. This is what these drugs do. It even says so on the warning labels. Guys go blind, lose part of their colon, have plastic surgeries to stuff silicone into their calves and under their cheekbones – it's a whole industry that rides codicil to the AIDS drug business."

A friend (of a friend) of mine tested HIV+ *twenty five years ago*, he refused all "medications" and he is still alive and well, which is very common among people who refuse the "medicines"! This recent article from *NaturalNews.com* entitled *"San Francisco woman proves that HIV doesn't always cause AIDS: no symptoms after 23 years"* makes the point very clear:

> "In the 23 years since she was diagnosed with HIV, 61-year-old Loreen Willenberg of Sacramento, Calif., has never taken any drugs to restrain the virus. She has never shown symptoms or become ill from HIV or AIDS. She has experienced no drop in her CD4 T-cells, the immune cells targeted by HIV.
>
> "I haven't had a decline of CD4 cell count at all, and that's pretty magnificent, and I'm very humbled by that," Willenberg said.
>
> "In a clinical sense, I'm not progressing towards AIDS," she said. "I'm not progressing towards the disease stage."

The article says that HIV doesn't *always* cause AIDS, but the simple truth is that it *never* causes AIDS! Ever!

What happens with people who die of AIDS is that they are

first; falsely diagnosed (misdiagnosed) with those shady, inaccurate HIV "tests", second; given toxic drugs that they don't need, which *destroy the immune system* and are *deadly toxic* beyond belief, and then third; **die**, not because of HIV, but because of liver failure and other factors from the toxic poison that "doctors" give them as "medicine"! False diagnosis>toxic drugs>death (not from AIDS but from the drugs). Those who refuse the drugs *keep living normal lives*!

6) As I mentioned above, Professor Duesberg accurately points out that HIV/AIDS cases have consistently remained in the same category of high risk groups: failing to spread into other areas of the population. If it's a "contagious virus" then it would be more evenly spread throughout the population, but it remains confined to 85% men and the two main high risk groups, gay males and IV drug users. This is not compatible behavior with the idea that it's a "contagious virus." If it was contagious then more women would be getting it, more teenagers would be getting it, more hospital workers would be getting it, more hemophiliacs would be getting it, etc.! But it remains contained within the same groups of people that it was in when they invented the term "AIDS" and has not spread to other areas of the population! "Contagious viruses" don't discriminate. If it was really a contagious virus it would be much more spread out by now, *but it's not*.

Conclusion) After years of researching the facts I have determined that the "HIV=AIDS" hypothesis was not a discovery but an *invention* by the government, the pharmaceutical industry and the medical industry working in collusion and then propagated by their mainstream media puppets for the purpose of increasing drug profits, among other reasons.

There is no hard science to back the bogus claim that HIV causes AIDS, even the "experts" will tell you that they don't know *how* HIV causes AIDS (but they'll never admit that it doesn't cause it at all!):

- "We are still very confused about the mechanisms that lead to CD4 T-cell depletion, but at least now we are *confused at a higher level of understanding.*" - Dr. Paul Johnson, *Harvard Medical School*

- "*We still do not know how*...the virus destroys CD4 + T-cells...Several hypothesis have been proposed to explain the loss of CD4 + T-cells, *some of which seem to be diametrically opposed."* - Joseph McCune, Immunologist

- "Despite considerable advances in HIV science in the past 20 years, the reason why HIV-1 infection is pathogenic is still debated...There is a general misconception that more is known about HIV-1 than any other virus and that all of the important issues regarding HIV-1 biology and pathogenesis have been resolved. On the contrary, *what we know represents only a thin veneer on the surface of what needs to be known."* - Mario Stevenson, Virologist

- "Twenty-five years into the HIV epidemic, a complete understanding of what drives the decay of CD4 cells – the essential event of HIV disease – *is still lacking."* - W. Keith Henry, Pablo Tebas and H. Clifford Lane

- "Although 12 years have passed since the identification of HIV as the cause of AIDS, *we do not yet know* how HIV kills its target, the CD4 + T-cell, nor how this killing cripples the immune system." - T.H. Finkel, *National Jewish Center for Immunology and Respiratory Medicine*

31 years after it was announced that HIV causes AIDS, if you try to look up how HIV infects and kills T-cells, you'll find a big void. There is no evidence that HIV kills T-cells, as a matter of fact Professor Duesberg reported that HIV **did not** kill T-cells in laboratory petri dishes, and I haven't seen anyone prove otherwise.

There is no real definition of what "AIDS" is, and there is no scientific evidence at all to demonstrate that the live HIV virus has ever infected the blood of a human being. There has been no true isolation of the virus, no electron microscope pictures of HIV in the blood of a patient, and the "tests" for HIV are admitted *by the manufacturers* to be *insufficient for diagnosing HIV infection.* Even the man who **invented the PCR test**, Dr. Kerry Mullis, adamantly states that HIV is not the cause of AIDS. All of this while at the same time "treatments" have become a *multi-billion dollar industry.* The so-called "AIDS Virus" is a scam and the "treatments" for it kill people unnecessarily!

Cancer: The Numerous Forbidden Cures

"Everyone should know that most cancer research is largely a fraud…"

- Linus Pauling Ph.D. (1901-1994) Two time Nobel Prize winner.

Welcome to the longest chapter of this book. The *reason* that this is the longest chapter is that cancer is the biggest fraud in the history of mainstream "medicine" and has killed millions of people basically for no reason. **Cancer is very curable** and there are *many* effective treatments for cancer! That might be hard for you to believe if you've been stuck in the mainstream all your life, watching and reading the mainstream "news", listening to mainstream "doctors", listening to mainstream "scientists", listening to the government's lies, and believing as you're ordered and instructed to believe by society and the people who work to **suppress** these cures in order to rake in billions in profits every year on their so-called "treatments". Yes, it might be real hard for you to believe that there are so many proven safe and effective treatments for cancer if you buy into mainstream propaganda hook, line and sinker. But I've got news for you; the mainstream is a *monumental lie*. You've been had. You've been duped. You've been made a fool of. You've been victimized. You've been shat on. *They lie*. They teach "knowledge" in their institutions that isn't true, and that "knowledge" is accepted by most people in society as fact, but it's not. It's *bullshit*. If you're rolling your eyes right now I challenge you to *keep reading*. **You'll see**. Just keep reading.

Cancer. Everybody knows someone who has died from it. If you don't have a family member who has died from it, you most certainly do know someone who has. Cancer is an epidemic. Every year almost 10 million people worldwide are diagnosed with cancer, and some 7 million die from it. The USA, the home of the "greatest health care system in the world", ranks third on the list of countries where cancer is most prevalent. 100 years ago only 1 in 80 Americans were diagnosed with cancer. Today, with all of the genetically modified and chemical laden "foods", fluoride and chlorine in our drinking water, chemicals in the air that we breathe, etc. the rate of cancer has increased to 1 in 3. Amazing isn't it? One out of every **three** people alive will be diagnosed with cancer. And that number is estimated to increase to *1 in 2* by the year 2020.

According to the *World Health Organization* (WHO), cancer rates are estimated to increase by 50% over the course of the next 15 years.

The *War on Cancer* was officially signed into law in 1971 by "Tricky Dicky, I am not a crook" Nixon. Ever since then it has been a no-win war, with the "cure" always right around the corner, but never admitted to be found.

Dr. Richard Day, the head of *Planned Parenthood*, addressed a meeting of doctors in Pittsburgh in 1969:

> "We can cure almost every cancer right now. Information is on file in the Rockefeller Institute, if it's ever decided that it should be released."

Day said that letting people die of cancer would slow down population growth.

> "You may as well die of cancer as something else."

Cancer is a quagmire, like Viet Nam. And of course, it was *designed* that way for the benefit of the drug profiteers. That's how they operate. Once you figure out their standard "modus operandi" it makes all the sense in the world. Can you think of a better plan to continue rolling in the revenue? I can't. And that's how they do things, not just for cancer, but for pretty much everything.

> "The Cancer Industry survives and thrives by perpetually searching for "the cure" but never finding it. This multi-billion dollar juggernaut is simply not interested in finding a cure, unless that cure consists of patented drugs that can be sold at a premium and need to be taken for the rest of the patient's life, thus creating a perpetual "revenue stream". So, in all actuality, the Cancer Industry is perpetuating lies and fraud. This fraud is of unspeakable magnitude, it has spanned more than a century, and it has unnecessarily caused the premature deaths of tens of millions of people."

> - Ty Bollinger in his book *Cancer: Step Outside the Box*

The sad thing about that is that the *vast majority* of deaths from cancer are totally and completely unnecessary. Even the latest stages of cancer have been cured, again and again and again and again. There are *numerous* natural treatments for cancer that are proven to be very effective, and I'll get to those very soon.

But first; what is cancer? Most people don't understand what it really is. They think it's a complicated disease. They aren't aware of the fact that *all people* develop cancerous cells in their body on a routine basis. Quite literally *everyone* "has cancer". It's a normal, every day thing. It's a process of cell multiplication that gets out of hand and takes over, unless, of course, you have a good, strong *immune system*. The *immune system* keeps the cancerous cells from multiplying, spreading and taking over, and there are numerous herbs that assist the immune system and give it a powerful boost (see the *Common Cold* section for information on those). Sadly, "doctors" today provide toxic "treatments" that *break down* the immune system, rather than make it stronger. Their standard methods quite *literally promote cancer* and death. Mainstream "medicine" is killing people left and right, unnecessarily. Is this a crime against humanity? That's an understatement. Hitler killed six million Jews. The medical industry has killed hundreds of millions with their drugs, their bogus "treatments" and the suppression of cures for cancer.

The Cancer Industry has three standard "treatments" for cancer, and they are all *very profitable*; Surgery, Chemotherapy and Radiation. **Cut, Poison and Burn!** All three are utter failures. These "treatments" are so worthless that if the patient lives for more than 5 years they call it a "cure". Their current "cure" rate, all combined and totaled together, is *only 3%!* No better than it was in the 1950s! And no better than it would be if people did nothing at all about their cancer! 3% is indeed pathetic, and that's an understatement. Think of all the billions spent since 1950 on so-called "research" and then think about the fact that the best they can come up with, supposedly, is cutting, poisoning and burning! *The cancer industry is a fraud.*

Chemotherapy and radiation are proven carcinogens (*cause cancer!*). Why would anyone be so dumb as to believe that poisoning the body and destroying the immune system with toxic shit would help something? When you have cancer you need to *build* the immune system because it's then that you *need it more than ever*! But for some reason people believe that just because a "doctor" told them that chemotherapy and radiation are "what's best" they'll argue 'til they're blue in the face and then they'll allow themselves to be murdered by "medical professionals" because they irrationally have blind faith and trust the so-called "healthcare" system! Common sense here is optional, apparently, even when their own lives are at stake! Again; *"Beam me up Scotty, there's no intelligent life on this planet."* But that's the standard practice of the Cancer Industry, murdering people with poisons, and millions of people quite literally ***buy*** into it, spending tens, even hundreds of thousands *per patient* for "treatments" that are worthless and *kill them dead* while the Cancer Industry rakes in billions and billions of dollars annually because of it. There is only one thing that keeps these murdering criminals in business, and that is the ignorance of the people. With properly educated masses, we could put the Medical Mafia out of business, and that's the main purpose of me writing this book. To *educate*.

When we consider the standard methods, surgery seems to make sense, right? It sounds good. Removing the tumor would help wouldn't it? Well, no. Not really. First of all, by the time cancer is typically detected close to 100% of all cancer patients already have cancerous cells *in their blood*, which makes it totally worthless to try and cut out a tumor and then say "we got it all". Bullshit! *It's still in their blood*! Additionally, cancer surgeries and biopsies often spread the cancer even more by spilling millions of cancer cells into the patient's blood also, and with the exception of some very minor forms of cancer, the average survival rate after cancer surgeries is only 1 year and 5 months (about the same as doing nothing at all). Even minor skin cancers are known to keep coming back after they've been surgically removed, and that's because the Cancer Industry doesn't address the *root of the problem,* they address the symptoms, which obviously doesn't work, based upon their results. They keep mutilating people left and right, and less than 3% of them live longer than 5 years afterwards. But that's ok, it's makes them money, and that's what counts right? I hate to sound repetitive, but they don't care because they roll in *$200 billion* per year, and that's their goal, not saving people. You can call me cynical, but I'm simply pointing out the truth and calling it what it is; mass murder for profit.

Fact; chemotherapy drugs originate from nitrogen mustard gas experiments during World Wars I and II. The Geneva Conventions have outlawed the use of mustard gas in wars, but they still give it to cancer patients! They saw that mustard gas destroyed fast growing tissue and that gave them ideas. They decided to try it with cancer. They were right about one thing, chemotherapy drugs can and do destroy cancerous tissue and shrink tumors, but chemotherapy drugs are *highly toxic*, like the drug AZT that I mentioned in the section about AIDS. They destroy the immune system, *cause cancer,* destroy red blood cells and kill vital organs.

> "Most cancer patients in this country die from chemotherapy. Chemotherapy does not eliminate breast, colon, or lung cancers. This fact has been documented for over a decade, yet doctors still use chemotherapy for these tumors."

> - Dr. Allen Levin

Just like "AIDS" patients, most cancer patients die from the *"treatment"* unnecessarily! In rare cases, chemotherapy might buy the patient a little bit more time, but it's not *quality* time. I'm sure you're aware of the effects of chemotherapy. Your hair falls out, you're nauseated, you vomit, you're dizzy, you get headaches, etc. Sure, it destroys cancer cells, but *clearly* this isn't a healthy method. I personally would rather die of cancer than be administered poison like chemotherapy.

> "Treating cancer with chemotherapy is like treating alcoholism with vodka...Cancer cannot be cured by the very thing that causes it. Don't let some cancer doctor talk you into chemotherapy using his fear tactics. They're good at that. So next time he insists that you take some chemotherapy, **ask him to drink some first**. If your oncologist isn't willing to drink chemotherapy to prove it's safe, why on earth would you agree to have it injected in your body?"

> - Mike Adams of *NaturalNews.com*

A recent article from *NYDailyNews.com* entitled *"Shock study: Chemotherapy can backfire, make cancer worse by triggering tumor growth"* reveals other interesting information:

> "Scientists found that healthy cells damaged by chemotherapy secreted more of a protein called WNT16B, which boosts cancer cell survival. 'The increase in WNT16B was completely unexpected,' said Peter Nelson, of the Fred Hutchinson Cancer Research Center (in Seattle, WA)."

> **Full article is here**: *http://www.nydailynews.com/life-style/health/shock-study-chemotherapy-backfire-cancer-worse-triggering-tumor-growth-article-1.1129897*

And from *PubMed.gov* we have a study entitled *"The contribution of cytotoxic chemotherapy to 5-year survival in adult malignancies"*:

> "RESULTS: The overall contribution of curative and adjuvant cytotoxic chemotherapy to 5-year survival in adults was estimated to be 2.3% in Australia and 2.1% in the USA."

> **Full article is here**: *http://www.ncbi.nlm.nih.gov/pubmed/15630849*

Just barely over 2% of chemo patients live longer than 5 years! Very pathetic indeed! *Poison* simply isn't medicine, plain and simple.

> "As a chemist trained to interpret data, it is incomprehensible to me that physicians can ignore the clear evidence that chemotherapy does much, much more harm than good."

- Dr. Alan C. Nixon, former President of the *American Chemical Society*

It baffles my mind as to why so many people are willing to submit to these so-called "treatments"! I assume it's because they believe it's their only choice, but like I already said, even if it was my only choice, I personally would rather just die of cancer. As a matter of fact, *roughly 75% of all doctors* would never submit to chemotherapy themselves. Dr. Charles Mathe, a French cancer specialist said:

> "If I contracted cancer, I would never go to a standard cancer treatment center. Only cancer victims who live far from such centers have a chance."

Dr. Glenn Warner, who passed away in the year 2000, was a highly successful alternative cancer specialist. He had this to say about it:

> "We have a multi-billion dollar industry that is killing people, right and left, just for financial gain. Their idea of research is to see whether two doses of this poison is better than three doses of that poison."

In a study conducted at the *McGill Cancer Center* in Montreal, considered one of the best cancer centers in the world, they asked 64 oncologists if they would submit to chemotherapy if they were diagnosed with cancer. **58 *of them said no*.** Their most general reasons were because chemotherapy drugs don't work and because they are toxic to the system. So here we have **91%** of the oncologists surveyed at one of the "greatest cancer centers in the world" saying "No way!" to chemotherapy, but of course, they keep on giving it to patients *anyway*, because like I keep saying, a very high percentage of "doctors" are only interested in the money, not curing disease. They blindly do as they're told by their masters (the drug companies) and reap their financial rewards, enjoy trips to the Bahamas, etc. I personally can't comprehend how they're able to sleep at night, but then again, I believe in common decency.

> "I've met one oncologist in my life who wouldn't be classified as a sociopath...they are willing to give chemicals to a person, knowing they won't help the person...knowing that it causes harm, collecting the money for it, and moving on to the next patient, and that by definition would make them sociopathic. No conscience, no remorse, yet giving them drugs they themselves would never take...I know there are exceptions but I've only ever met one, in 30 years...she was the only one with a conscience."

- Dr. Michael Farley

A former Vice President of the *American Cancer Society*,

Dr. John Laszlo states in his book entitled *Understanding Cancer* that secondary tumors are *25 times* more likely to occur when chemotherapy and radiation are given together.

Concerning radiation "treatments", it's common knowledge among just about everybody that *radiation causes cancer.* Dr. Ralph Moss states in his book entitled *The Cancer Industry*:

> "In 1902, a German doctor recorded the first case of human cancer caused by radiation: the tumor had appeared on the site of a chronic ulceration caused by X-ray exposure. Experimental studies performed in 1906 suggest that leukemia (cancer of the blood) could be caused by exposure to the radioactive element radium. By 1911, 94 cases of radiation induced cancer had been reported, more than half of them (54) in doctors or technicians. By 1922, over 100 radiologists had died from X-ray-induced cancer...I had a brain cancer specialist sit in my living room and tell me that he would never take radiation if he had a brain tumor. And I asked him 'But do you send people for radiation?' and he said 'Of course, I'd be drummed out of the hospital if I didn't.'"

I personally could never allow myself to have such shitty morals. Yes, he was doing it to save his job, but even so, he was sending innocent, unsuspecting people off to die, knowing that they were going to die, knowing that the treatment would kill them. I'd rather be a dishwasher. I'd rather be homeless. No amount of money would make it ok for me to do that to people, but then again I have a *conscience.*

Concerning radiation and breast cancer:

> "Mammograms increase the risk for developing breast cancer and raise the risk of spreading or metastasizing an existing growth."

> - Dr. Charles Simone, former *National Cancer Institute* associate

In a Swedish study of 60,000 women, **70%** of tumors diagnosed by mammograms turned out to be **false positives**. In other words women are exposed to radiation that *significantly raises* their chances of getting cancer for a test that is *wrong 70% of the time*!

> "Regular mammography of younger women increases their cancer risks. Analysis of controlled trials over the last decade has shown consistent increases in breast cancer mortality within a few years of commencing screening. This confirms evidence of the high sensitivity of the premenopausal breast, and on cumulative carcinogenic effects of radiation."

> - Dr. Samuel Epstein in his book *The Politics of Cancer*

So why do they keep using mammograms if they're inaccurate and if they cause cancer? Follow the money trail! If a mammogram costs $100.00 a pop (they cost much more than that, but this is hypothetical) and every one of the *70 million* women over 40 has a mammogram every year, that comes to a *7 billion dollar* a year industry! Pretty easy to figure out when you know how they operate! Cynical? Nope. Just pointing to the truth and calling it what it is.

If they *really cared* about women's health, they could stop using mammograms *very easily*. There is no need for mammograms, they're far, *far* inferior to a technology called "thermography" which is 100% safe! Thermography also happens to detect tumors *years sooner* than either mammograms or physical exams. This is how it works; tissues that are *turning into tumors* are higher in temperature than healthy tissue, therefore all that is required to detect them is infra-red camera technology. Not only is it an accurate method of detection, it catches it *before* it has actually turned into a tumor:

> "Before tissue degenerates into cancer, the body's metabolic rate around the site increases. A unique aspect of cancerous tumor growth is a process called neo-angiogenesis (new blood vessel growth). As the cells multiply, they need an increase blood supply to bring in nutrients and remove waste. The increase in circulation gives off heat. An infra-red type camera can detect this heat, giving the patient and doctor an opportunity to take action long before a tumor develops. This makes thermography a tremendous weapon in the fight against breast cancer!"
>
> - Dr. Robert Rowen

But they don't use this technology much because it's nowhere near as profitable. They use mammograms, which cause cancer (which is good for repeat business, of course) and then women are given radiation for breast cancer, which brings in even more revenue.

> "Complications following high-dose radiotherapy for breast cancer are: fibrous, shrunken breasts, rib fractures, pleural and/or lung scarring, nerve damage, scarring around the heart...suppression of all blood cells, immune suppression...Many radiation complications do no occur for several years after treatment, giving the therapist and the patient a false sense of security for a year or two following therapy. The bone marrow, in which blood cells are made, is largely obliterated in the field of irradiation...This is an irreversible effect."
>
> - Dr. Robert F. Jones, *Seattle Times*, July 27, 1980

Clearly chemotherapy and radiation are antiproductive "treatments" but they make the Cancer Industry *billions of dollars* a year, so that's good enough then, right? A conscience? What's that?

In 1966, Dr. Irwin D. Bross and four colleagues wrote a series of articles entitled *"Is Toxicity Really Necessary?"* simply questioning whether or not it was possible to find *less toxic* treatments for cancer. The government *cut off their funding immediately.* In other words "don't make us look bad or we'll cut you off so fast it'll make your head spin". The Medical Mafia clearly works very hard to protect its multi-billion dollar empire, and anyone who messes with them gets the hammer.

There are numerous natural, side effect free treatments and proven cancer cures with great success rates out there, but you've probably never heard of them because the owners of Big Pharma control the media, and the medical schools, and the mainstream scientists, and they suppress all information that threatens their profits with thugs and guns. "How dare you discover a better way! That threatens our empire!"

"There have been many cancer cures, and all have been ruthlessly and systematically suppressed with a Gestapo-like thoroughness by the cancer establishment. The cancer establishment is the not-too-shadowy association of the American Cancer Society, the leading cancer hospitals, the National Cancer Institute and the FDA. The shadowy part is the fact that these respected institutions are very much dominated by members of the pharmaceutical industry, which profits so incredibly much from our profession-wide obsession with chemotherapy."

- Dr. Robert C. Atkins

Cancer is big business. Not only do they make profits on their "treatments" they make millions selling drugs to "treat" the problems *created by their "treatments"* (chemotherapy in particular). Cancer is a *money making machine*, and if the cure(s) got out to the public their party would be all over.

"Over the past century, hundreds of caring, concerned, and conscientious alternative doctors and herbalists have been treated like common criminals for the 'crime' of curing people of terminal diseases in an unapproved manner by heavy-handed government agents who swoop down on clinics with machine guns and body armor. All the while, these same agencies posture themselves before TV cameras and the public under the ludicrous pretense of being servants of the people and protectors of the common good."

- Ty Bollinger in his book *Cancer: Step Outside the Box*

In the book entitled *The Healing of Cancer* by Barry Lynes, he mentioned the documented fact that...

"...in 1953, a US Senate Investigation reported that a conspiracy existed to suppress effective cancer treatments. The Senator in charge of the investigation conveniently died. The investigation was halted. It was neither the first nor the last of a number of strange deaths involving people in positions to do damage to those running the nation's cancer program. For many years, the American Medical Association (AMA) and the American Cancer Society (ACS) coordinated their 'hit' lists of innovative cancer researchers who were to be ostracized."

Right now I'd like to tell you about those cures I keep

mentioning. I'll start with the ones that have faced the highest degree of merciless suppression by the Medical Mafia and their gangs of thugs.

"Any doctor in the United States who uses alternative methods to cure cancer will be destroyed. You cannot name me a doctor doing well with cancer using alternative therapies that is not under attack. And I know these people. I've interviewed them."

- Dr. Gary Null

The Persecution of Stanislaw R. Burzynski

Meet Dr. Burzynski, an internationally recognized physician and scientist from Lublin, Poland who has devoted his whole life to cancer research. In 1967 he discovered "antineoplastons" which are small peptides produced by the liver that control cell multiplication. Antineoplastons are naturally in the blood and urine of healthy people, but *not* in people with cancer. Logic suggests that maybe *putting them back* when they're missing would have a healing effect. Dr. Burzynski tried it and it works. He uses synthetically reproduced antineoplastons for his treatments. They quite literally turn off life processes in abnormal cells and force them to die without hurting normal cells.

Dr. Burzynski has cured over 50 kinds of cancer with antineoplastons, including breast, bladder, lung and terminal brain cancer. One form of cancer, childhood brainstem glioma, has never been cured before. Burzynski has done it dozens of times. His total success rate (for all cancers) has been nearly **60% over a 40 year period**, as compared to the Cancer Industry's incompetent 2% or 3%. And he doesn't use poison. Gee, what a concept!

The Cancer Industry's idea of a "cure" is if the patient lives for 5 years or longer after diagnosis. Dr. Burzynski has treated people *as children* who grew up to get married and have children, without ever seeing any more signs of cancer in either themselves or their children. They are cured for life and they go on to live normal, healthy lives. That *never* happens with chemo or radiation!

Various cancer survivors are presented in the films *Burzynski the Movie: Cancer Is Serious Business* (parts 1 and 2) who have been cured by this process, and they supply their medical records to support their claims. You can purchase the DVDs and read all about it at _BurzynskiMovie.com_. If you take the time to watch the films you'll see all the proof you need, there's no disputing the efficacy of antineoplastons based upon his results. Also, the book _Knockout: Interviews With Doctors Who Are Curing Cancer and How To Prevent Getting It In the First Place_ by Suzanne Somers features an excellent interview with Dr. Burzynski.

As should be expected by anyone who knows how the Medical Mafia operates, for the last 40 years Dr. Burzynski has been harassed, gagged, had funding cut off, been raided by the FDA, and has been threatened with _290 years in prison and 18.5 million in fines_ among other things, for the "crime" of curing cancer. The FDA's excuse for their harassment is that the good doctor is using cures that are not "approved" by them. You're only allowed to cure cancer if we say it's ok! How dare you cure cancer without our approval!

In any "great country" if they saw a doctor who was curing cancer, they'd give the man a medal, a Nobel Prize and make a hero out of him. That's the way it _should be_. In "great countries" they don't _hide_ the cure for cancer, they _celebrate it_ when it arrives! But in this country doctors who cure cancer get threatened with prison!

When the FDA tried to put Dr. Burzynski in jail, there were two federal trials. There were literally hundreds of people showing up for his support. Two-thirds were patients of his, the rest were family members of patients. Richard Jaffe, the health care attorney representing Dr. Burzynski, said:

> "In my twenty-five years practicing as a health care attorney, I have never seen a physician who has been subjected to to the unrelenting government persecution that Dr. Burzynski faced. Early on, the FDA tried and failed to obtain an injunction stopping him from treating terminally ill cancer patients. Between 1985 and 1995, Burzynski was investigated by four federal grand juries. The first three refused to indict him; the fourth did. Fortunately, the gods were smiling on us. We won the case and Dr. Burzynski was acquitted of all charges after two federal criminal trials...Congress held several hearings on FDA abuse in which the Burzynski persecution was front and center. Eventually, Congress forced the FDA to allow him to continue to treat all of his patients and to begin clinical trials. Throughout those dark days, the clinic's doors never closed, due largely to Burzynski's courage, patients, and maybe some pretty fair legal work."

Many former patients have come forward in courts testifying for him, saying that they would be dead if it wasn't for him and giving him credit for being the hero that he truly is. Dr.

Burzynski is winning the biggest legal battle against the FDA in US history, having escaped all prosecution because he has been properly going through the legal channels. He has *not broken a single law*, but he's still being harassed and the future of antineoplastons looks grim.

As of 2009 antineoplastons have completed Phase II FDA-supervised clinical trials, but the final phase of FDA clinical trials has a price tag of $300 million, which again shows how criminal the FDA is. They prevent these proven cancer cures (and there are many) from being "approved" by putting huge price tags on the FDA trials! Do you want your safe and effective cancer treatment approved? Ok then *give us a quarter of a billion dollars* and we might think about it! You would think that with such an amazing discovery the federal government would be throwing funds in Dr. Burzynski's direction making it real easy for him to get antineoplastons approved, **but no**. They're doing everything they can to block that from happening because they're a bunch of corrupt bastards who only care about one thing, drug company profits. The system guarantees that multi-billion dollar drug companies are pretty much the only ones who get approval, and if something like antineoplastons would hurt their profits, well then guess what? They'll never study it, much less try to get it approved. And so Dr. Burzynski is on his own trying to foot the huge bill for the approval on his miraculous cancer treatment while the government and the FDA work *against* him, meanwhile the "healthcare" industry keeps on poisoning people with chemo and radiation. Isn't that fucking incredible?

Excuse me, but if antineoplastons have successfully cured people over and over again, *which they have*, then *what the hell's the problem*? Chemotherapy *kills hundreds of thousands* of people per year because it is highly *ineffective*, yet *it's approved* (because it's very, very profitable!) but the safe and side effect free treatments of this great doctor still haven't been approved!? Something is very, very wrong here! This is just totally unacceptable!

Dr. Burzynski was *banned* from using antineoplastons (again!) in 2013, but has since had the sanctions lifted as of June 23rd 2014. The following is from the *BurzynskiMovie.com*:

"The Burzynski Research Institute, Inc. (BRI) announced today that U.S. Food and Drug Administration (FDA) has notified the company that its partial clinical hold on its IND for Antineoplastons A10/AS2-1 Injections has been lifted. The FDA has determined that under its IND the Company may initiate its planned Phase 3 study in newly diagnosed diffuse, intrinsic, brainstem glioma. The Company is continuing discussions with the Agency in an effort to finalize additional details of the phase 3 study protocol for the potential clinical trial."

Full article is here: http://www.burzynskimovie.com/index.php/component/content/article/158#.VTs6OCFVikp

Antineoplastons have still not been approved and it has been nearly 50 years since their discovery. Very, very dark forces are in control of the medical system in this country and "we the people" have to stand up to them! I hate to keep repeating myself (wait, no I don't!) but the reason that effective cancer treatments are being suppressed is really quite simple; it's the the *profits first, people last* system that is in place, not only for health care but for everything else, too. As long as people have the power to make a quick buck off of other people's misfortune (in this case getting cancer), then they'll do it, because the *profit based system* that is in place today encourages dog eat dog competition; it encourages people to walk all over each other in the name of money, which is absolutely *anti-productive* for the human race because anything that could potentially hurt the profits of large industries gets suppressed, not only in health care but in *everything*, and the majority of the people suffer because of it. The most *consistent* thing about capitalism is *corruption*. Period. You can *always* count on rampant corruption when you're dealing with a system that places profits as the top priority. How **immoral** is it, how **evil** is it to profit off of someone's poor health (cancer) while you give them inferior treatments (chemotherapy, radiation, surgery) and watch them die because giving them genuinely effective treatments would cut into your profits? Think about that question for a while.

Five Years in Prison for Selling Apricot Seeds

Meet Jason Vale, a *World Champion Arm Wrestler* from New York. Jason has been battling cancer since 1986 at the age of 18, when he was diagnosed with a very rare type of cancer called an "Askin's Tumor". When he was diagnosed there had only been 20 reported cases of this particular type of cancer and it had a

100% death rate.

The tumor, about the size of a grapefruit, was between his back and ribs and was causing fluid to build up in his lungs. He opted for surgery. As is typical with surgery for cancer, within one year the tumor came back much worse than before and he could hardly walk as the tumor was affecting his spinal cord. Again, he had surgery, this time opting for chemo and radiation as well, nearly dying from the toxicity in the process.

For seven miraculous years he had no problems with cancer, but then...

> "...during a routine scan, as I was taking 40 Tylenol # 4 with codeine per day it was discovered that I had a tumor in my kidney. I told the doctor my thoughts were that all the medication I was taking was the direct cause of the tumor. He found this theory to be silly. Upon research, I found that pain killers have been proven to cause kidney carcinomas, which was what I had. He disagreed completely. Later, it was shown through various tests, that the tumor in my kidney was malignant. It was about to start all over again. I went to the kidney specialist who said I had to get my kidney taken out. Yet the more questions I asked him, the more aggravated he got. I simply wanted to know as much as possible about my disease so I could be in a position to make an educated decision. I left his office, returned once, and then never again. I received subsequent certified letters from his office warning me of the dangers I was in if left untreated. It was fun making paper planes out of them."

Shortly thereafter, a friend from church gave Jason a VHS tape of *World Without Cancer* by G. Edward Griffin. This documentary is based upon the work of Dr. Ernst T. Krebs who, in the 1950s, developed a theory that cancer is caused by a deficiency in "nitrilosides", a substance found in over 1200 plants including apricots, peaches, apples, bean sprouts and more. Dr. Krebs extracted the nitrilosides and developed a drug with it that he named *Laetrile*. Eventually the naturally occurring substance became known as *Amygdalin* or *Vitamin B17*. The drug was never approved by the FDA, but of course, the natural substance remained which can be purchased at just about any health food store or supermarket.

Like almost all doctors who publicize effective cancer treatments, Dr. Krebs had his own problems:

> "After presenting a rather effective lecture on cancer...the windshield was shot out of my car on the road back to San Francisco. The next night the glass window in the tail gate was shot out (300 miles removed from the first shooting). The police said 'maybe somebody is trying to tell you something'. The late Arthur Harris, M.D. was threatened by two men with assassination if he continued to use laetrile. Since that time we have decentralized the work so that, if any two of us are shot out of the saddle, it will only have a slight negative effect on the program."

G. Edward Griffin's film inspired Jason to start eating *apricot seeds* on a regular basis and as a result, his cancer started *disappearing*. Amazing isn't it, that something as simple as apricot seeds can hold cancer in check and keep it at bay? Jason's been doing it since 1993.

> "I had cancer three times, the first time when I was eighteen years old, the second time at 19 and then 15 years ago at 26. Since the last time, I've been eating the apricot seeds as my only therapy along with some basic diet changes. The first time I was operated on and the second time, a combination of operation, chemo, radiation and small diet changes....but the third time...APRICOT SEEDS and apricot seeds only! Found in over 1200 foods, which we don't eat anymore in our culture, the components of the apricot seed make it nearly impossible for cancer to grow in a body free of cancer. For a person that has cancer, there are many different scenarios however, start eating the seeds immediately, weather or not you are doing chemo and radiation."

Jason has been watching his tumor shrink as he eats the apricot seeds, and enlarge when he's not eating them very much, which is the standard correlation seen when people start using amygdalin.

Amygdalin molecules contain one part hydrogen cyanide, one part benzaldehyde and two parts glucose. I know what you must be thinking at this point, "cyanide!?" Yes, well, first of all, the cyanide content is harmless unless it is released from the molecule. In order for the cyanide to be released from the molecule it has to come into contact with one enzyme in particular, and that enzyme is called beta-glucosidase. Conveniently, beta-glucosidase is *only contained in cancerous cells*, not in normal cells! So when the amygdalin molecules come in contact with the cancerous cells, the beta-glucosidase in those cancerous cells unlocks the cyanide and the benzaldehyde (which is also toxic to cancer) and it quite literally kills off the cancerous cells. Additionally, the synergistic combination of the cyanide and the benzaldehyde makes both substances 100 times stronger than they would be by themselves. I'm sure you're wondering what impact this has on normal cells? Well, normal cells contain a *protective enzyme* called rhodanese. Rhodanese does, in fact, *neutralize* the cyanide and benzaldehyde rendering them harmless to normal cells. In other words, there's no truth in the myth that says apricot seeds are poisonous. They are poisonous to *cancer cells only*. Chemotherapy, on the other hand, is *toxic to all cells*, and is proven to do more harm than good for patients.

Dr. Dean Burk, the former head of the Cytochemistry Department of the *National Cancer Institute*, clinically tested amygdalin personally.

"When we add laetrile (amygdalin) to a cancer culture under the microscope, providing the enzyme glucosidase also is present, we can see the cancer cells dying off like flies."

The Medical Mafia, in the pursuit of the protection of their beloved profits, has put many myths out there about the cyanide contained in amygdalin, warning people that it is "poisonous". That couldn't be farther from the truth! There is a population of people near Pakistan in the kingdom of Hunza that eat 200 times more amygdalin than Americans and they routinely eat the seeds from apricots. Visiting medical teams didn't find one case of cancer, their average life span is 85 and they are generally mentally alert all their lives as well. People who take chemotherapy, on the other hand, usually die quickly and have no quality of life either, being sick most of the time until they finally die. The Cancer Industry will put out "warnings" about Amygdalin trying to discourage people from using it, but of course chemotherapy is just fine, right? Not! But it makes them *money*.

Once Jason had his cancer under control with amygdalin (apricot seeds) he felt compelled to yell from rooftops and tell the world about his discovery. Jason was featured on a national television show called *Extra* appearing as "a world class arm wrestler who cured himself of cancer with apricot seeds", and it got such a popular response that they re-aired it. After all of the media attention and publicity he opened a website and began blogging about his personal cancer experience and amazing apricot seed discovery, also sending out mass emails to thousands of people with the subject line *"The Answer to Cancer is Known"*.

Eventually, Jason began selling apricot seeds on his website and worked up to about 28,000 customers world wide. He received thousands of emails from people thanking him and telling him how it had stopped their cancers from growing and spreading.

Apparently the Cancer Industry deemed Jason a threat to their precious profits because despite the fact that apricots are perfectly legal, and despite the fact that Jason had no complaints from any of his customers and despite the fact that his products were making it possible for thousands of people to be living lives with no worries of cancer, the FDA didn't like that because on Oct. 28th, 1998 they sent Jason a three page "warning letter" highlighting his *"promotion and distribution of the unapproved drug Laetrile in the form of apricot seeds, Vitamin B17 tablets and 'amygdalina' ampoules"* all of which are natural derivatives of apricots seeds.

Eventually Jason signed a statement saying that he would no longer promote his seeds as a "cancer cure" because the highly inappropriate and immoral law in the USA states that if you sell natural supplements you cannot make health claims on them, even if those claims are backed by numerous scientific studies (amygdalin is backed by science, as you will see in the next section). All health food stores and distributors are gagged from telling people about the health benefits of various supplements, and the reason for that is, of course, because they want to suppress that information because if the public had the info *it would cut into their drug profits*. So Jason simply started following that law. He was warned, signed a statement saying that he wouldn't make health claims, and then continued his business legally, no longer calling his product a "cancer cure". The statement that he signed *did not specify* that he had to stop selling his products. It seems to me that if they wanted him to stop selling any of his products that they should have *told him so*, right? But they *did not*.

Shortly thereafter, without any other warnings being made, the FDA raided Jason's home, seized his apricot seeds and computers and put Jason in jail. His bail was set at **$800,000** and on July 14th, 2003 Jason was sentenced to 63 months in *New York State Penitentiary*.

So let's get this straight; Big Pharma is permitted by the FDA to sell drugs that even the FDA admits *kill over 100,000 people per year*, but the products that Jason sold, which helped thousands of people effectively combat their cancers without side effects, are forbidden and he gets locked up in prison for five years for selling them! The FDA promotes chemotherapy which kills hundreds of thousands of people per year and only has a 2.1% success rate, but the FDA has a problem with *apricot seeds*! What a load of nonsense! Again, in a great country, if a cancer cure or effective treatment was discovered, especially one that is as safe and effective as this, they wouldn't hide it, they'd welcome it, and they'd treat the discoverer like a hero. Jason might not have discovered this cancer treatment, but he was a hero for educating so many people about it and saving so many people's lives.

While he was in prison his cancer got worse because he couldn't access his medicine. His mother would sneak him apricot seeds from time to time (in containers of nuts, because they look just like nuts), but he wasn't able to get as much as he needed. When he came out of prison on April 15th, 2008 his tumor had enlarged significantly but he's been holding it in check with his favorite medicine, apricot seeds! He still runs his website to this very day and he has apparently obtained permission to sell apricot products again because there are many products available for purchase. To purchase his products or to read more about his story go to *ApricotsFromGod.info*.

Fired For NOT Lying About Laetrile

Meet Ralph Moss, Ph.D., former Science Writer and Assistant Director of Public Affairs for one of the most prestigious and well known cancer centers in the world, *Memorial Sloan-Kettering Cancer Center,* from 1974 to 1977. A very large part of Ralph's job was to write press releases for the hospital about new developments in science regarding cancer, as well as handle calls from people with questions about cancer and various treatments.

During the course of writing one of his articles, Mr. Moss interviewed one of the scientists at the hospital, Dr. Kanematsu Sugiura, who was one of the world's premier cancer researchers at the time. The scientist informed Mr. Moss that he had seen repetitive and conclusive positive results over the course of two years of study while studying "amygdalin", otherwise known as Laetrile, the anticancer ingredient in *apricot seeds*. Sugiura concluded that Laetrile:

1) Inhibited the growth of tumors
2) Stopped the spreading of cancer in mice
3) Relieved pain
4) Acted as a cancer preventative
5) Improved general health

After receiving this information Mr. Moss got very excited and planned on writing a big report on it. He then went to his superiors with the good news. It was then that he got, as he puts it in his own words, the "shock of my life".

His superiors demanded that he cease and desist writing the story, saying that Dr. Sugiura's work was invalid, denying that it was real evidence. As the icing on the cake they proceeded to instruct Mr. Moss to write an article and press release for all major news stations stating that amygdalin was *worthless for cancer treatment*, in other words, they ordered him to lie through his teeth and report the exact opposite of the truth to the American people.

> "Certainly one story that needs to be told is that of Dr. Kanematsu Sugiura. In 1975, Dr. Sugiura was, and had been for some years, one of the most respected cancer research scientists at Sloan-Kettering. In working with cancerous mice, Dr. Sugiura found that, when he used Laetrile on these mice, seventy-seven per cent of them did not develop a spread of their disease (metastatic carcinoma). He repeated this study over and over for two years. The results were always the same. Dr. Sugiura took his findings to his superiors at Sloan-Kettering, but his study was never published. Instead, Sloan-Kettering published the results of someone else who claimed that he had used Dr. Sugiura's protocol. This 'someone else's study showed that there were no beneficial effects from the use of Laetrile. Dr. Sugiura complained. He was fired. A book was written about all of this entitled *The Anatomy of A Cover-up*. This book has all the actual results of Dr. Sugiura's work. These results do, indeed, show the benefit of Laetrile. Dr. Sugiura stated in this book, 'It is still my belief that Amygdalin cures metastases.' Amygdalin is, of course, the scientific name for Laetrile."
>
> - Philip E. Binzel, Jr., M.D. in his book *Alive and Well: One Doctor's Experience With Nutrition in the Treatment of Cancer Patients*

For the next few months Mr. Moss avoided the subject, and didn't write anything about amygdalin. He decided instead to take that time to conduct an investigation into the people he was working for. Who were they? Why were they asking him to lie? What was their incentive to cover-up such great news concerning cancer treatment? He discovered many interesting facts; their Board of Directors were investors in petrochemicals and CEO's of *top drug companies*, the Chairman and President of *Bristol-Meyers Squibb*, the world's biggest seller of *chemotherapy drugs* was also on the board. Seven of the nine members of the hospital's *Institutional Policy Committee* had ties to the *pharmaceutical industry* and the hospital itself invested in the *stock of those same drug companies*. Directors of the biggest tobacco companies in America, *Phillip Morris* and *RJR Nabisco* were also on the Board of Directors at the hospital and six directors also served on the boards of the *New York Times*, *CBS*, *Warner Communications*, *Reader's Digest* and other mainstream media outlets. In other words, the entire Board of Directors at one of the "world's premier cancer centers" was swimming in corruption and conflicts of interest, to say the very least. I'd love to report that this was an isolated case. I'd love to be able to say that it was only this hospital, but that simply wouldn't be the truth. The truth of the matter is that the entire industry functions that way and those procedures are standard practice. This incident at *Sloan-Kettering* was just another typical scenario in the Cancer Industry. Business as usual.

Mr. Moss wasn't able to avoid the subject of Amygdalin/Laetrile for very long. His secretary's phone was ringing off the hook with people wanting information about it, and again he was told to cover up the truth. He decided, after a conference with his family at home, that he was not willing to lie on behalf of the hospital. In November, 1977 he stood up at a press conference and "blew the whistle on *Memorial Sloan-Kettering Cancer Center*'s suppression of positive results with Laetrile". When he returned to the office he found that all of his files were padlocked, he was then escorted out of the building by two armed guards.

Mr. Moss considers that entire ordeal to have been a stepping stone that led the way to what he was truly meant to do in life; rather than working on the Board of Directors at a place like *Sloan-Kettering*, he has gone on to write 12 books, 3 documentaries and numerous articles in medical journals concerning complimentary and "alternative" cancer treatments. He eventually wrote a book about his laetrile experience entitled *Doctored Results: The Suppression of Laetrile at Sloan-Kettering Institute for Cancer Research*. He also runs the website *Cancer Decisions: The Moss Reports* which can be found at *CancerDecisions.com*.

<u>Arrested Over 200 Times for Curing Cancer</u>

Meet Harry Hoxsey, renowned herbalist and owner of the largest privately ran cancer treatment center in the USA during the 1950s, with over 17 branches nationwide. He opened his first cancer center in 1924, expanded quickly and cured thousands of people of cancer during his 30 years in business.

The story goes that John Hoxsey, Harry's grandfather, once had a horse that had cancer. He noticed that after getting cancer this horse would always graze around a certain area of the pasture where a certain kind of plants grew, plants that normally the horses wouldn't eat. Eventually, as the story goes, due to eating those specific plants, the horse was cancer free. I don't know how true that part of the story is, it sounds like a legend to me, but it doesn't matter if it's true or not because Harry's grandfather did in fact develop an herbal formula that he treated sick horses with. He had great success. When he passed away the formula was passed down to Harry's dad, who started treating humans with it. Harry eventually became the member of the family to use the formula on a large scale basis, having great success at curing many thousands of people from cancer.

The Hoxsey internal tonic consists of:

- Barberry Root
- Buckthorn Bark
- Burdock Root
- Cascara Sagrada
- Licorice Root
- Poke Berries and Root
- Potassium Iodide
- Prickly Ash Bark
- Red Clover Blossoms
- Stillingia Root

He stated that tomatoes, alcohol, processed flour and vinegar could possibly negate the formula's effects and advised against consuming those while on the program.

Harry Hoxsey was a very outgoing and confident person. He went on TV to advertise his clinics, and when he faced criticism he'd publicly challenge the medical authorities to come to his clinic and prove him wrong.

> "All I want is to have them come here – the American Medical Association, the Pure Food and Drug Administration, the Federal Government, anybody – come here and make an investigation and if I do not prove to them beyond any question of a doubt that our

treatment is superior to radium x-ray and surgery then I will lock the doors of this institution forever."

Of course they never accepted the challenge. Instead they continually harassed him, and had him arrested more than 200 times for "practicing medicine without a license".

District Attorney Al Templeton, perhaps Harry's biggest critic, had him arrested more than 100 times, that is until his brother developed cancer and was cured at one of Harry's clinics. He had tried chemotherapy and radiation without success. He then secretly went to Harry and was cured. Al Templeton was so moved by it that he went from continually prosecuting Harry to becoming his Defense Attorney!

In 1954 an independent team of 10 physicians visited Harry's clinic in Dallas for a two day inspection. They reviewed case histories, medical records and spoke with patients. At the end of their visit they issued an official statement declaring that the clinic was *"successfully treating pathologically proven cases of cancer, both internal and external, without the use of surgery, radium or x-ray"*.

At one point, Morris Fishbein, the head of the *American Medical Association*, who was also the editor of the *Journal of the American Medical Association*, tried to purchase the rights to Harry's herbal formula. If that isn't an *admission* that Harry's formula was effective then what is? If it didn't work then why would they be so worried about it and want to purchase it? The bottom line is that *it worked* and it was taking business away from them! They knew that if Harry's clinics got too big it would *destroy their entire cancer empire*, but their attempt to get the formula from Harry was met by a flat **no way**. Harry wasn't a sucker. He knew that if he sold them the formula it would never see the light of day again, it would be tucked away and hidden forever. He knew that the only reason they'd want to buy it from him was to *eliminate their competition*. He didn't fall for it. Harry was an honest man who wasn't interested in making money from his formula. He already had money, he was an oil millionaire, and he treated *everyone* who came to his clinics *regardless of their ability to pay*. He didn't want people to go without his treatments, he wanted to *help people*, therefore he *rejected* the offer to sell it.

From that point forward Fishbein put out articles in the

medical journals insulting his herbal formula calling it "worthless weeds" and basically slandering him every chance he got. A massive smear campaign was launched against Harry because if they couldn't buy him out they'd have to do it by any other means necessary. (Below is an actual flyer put out by the FDA during their smear campaign.)

Eventually Harry became known as "the biggest cancer quack of the century" due to their lies and accusations. Harry sued Morris Fishbein for slander and won, forcing him to resign from the *American Medical Association*, but the damage done to Harry's clinics was too much to repair. Harry eventually closed down all of his clinics and moved his main clinic to Tijuana, Mexico. Harry passed away in 1974 but his clinic is still open to this very day under new proprietorship. It's called the *Hoxsey Biomedical Center* and their website is at *HoxseyBioMedical.com*.

Public Beware!

WARNING AGAINST THE HOXSEY CANCER TREATMENT

Sufferers from cancer, their families, physicians, and all concerned with the care of cancer patients are hereby advised and warned that the Hoxsey treatment for internal cancer has been found worthless by two Federal courts.

The Hoxsey treatment costs $400, plus $60 in additional fees—expenditures which will yield nothing of value in the care of cancer. It consists essentially of simple drugs which are worthless for treating cancer.

The Food and Drug Administration conducted a thorough investigation of the Hoxsey treatment and the cases which were claimed to be cured. Not a single verified cure of internal cancer by this treatment has been found.

Those afflicted with cancer are warned not to be misled by the false promise that the Hoxsey cancer treatment will cure or alleviate their condition. Cancer can be cured only through surgery or radiation. Death from cancer is inevitable when cancer patients fail to obtain proper medical treatment because of the lure of a painless cure "without the use of surgery, x-ray, or radium" as claimed by Hoxsey.

Anyone planning to try this treatment should get the facts about it.

For further information write to:
U. S. DEPARTMENT OF HEALTH, EDUCATION, AND WELFARE
Food and Drug Administration
Washington 25, D. C.

The Suppression of Rene Caisse's Essiac Tea

Meet Rene Caisse, a nurse from Canada. In 1922 Rene was tending to one of her patients when she noticed some scar tissue on the lady's breast. The woman informed her that it used to be breast cancer, but was miraculously healed by an Indian Medicine Man, from the Ojibwa tribe, with an herbal tea. Eventually that woman gave the herbal tea formula to Rene who named it "Essiac" which is her last named spelled backwards.

Two years later Rene's aunt developed cancer. She decided to take the opportunity to test the tea on a cancer patient. After obtaining permission from her aunt's doctor Rene started giving her the tea. After approximately two months of drinking the tea three times daily, her aunt was cured and went on to live for 20 more years. Rene's mother was cured of her liver cancer as well, living for another 18 years!

Rene eventually opened up a clinic and cured thousands of people from various cancers for little or no fee. Most of her patients were people that had been through the mainstream medical system and had been told they were going to die. They were coming to her for "last chance" treatments. Rene gave treatments of Essiac both orally and intravenously. The vast majority of those that had no damage to major organs survived and lived long normal lives, but of course, there were some who didn't make it. All in all, her success rates were far superior to anything the medical establishment was doing, and most of her patients were experiencing miraculous recoveries.

In 1937 Rene was contacted by Dr. John Wolfer, the director of a tumor clinic at *Northwestern University Medical School* in Chicago, IL. He wanted to do clinical trials and arranged for 30 terminal cancer patients to be treated with Essiac Tea under the supervision of five doctors. Rene agreed and crossed the border into the US with her bottles of Essiac Tea. After 18 months of trials, the supervising team of doctors concluded that Essiac Tea *"prolonged life, shrank tumors, and reduced pain"*.

Meanwhile back home Rene had been treating up to 600 people per week at her clinic and the outstanding success of her treatments eventually caught the attention of the *Canadian Ministry of Health and Welfare* and the *Canadian Parliament*. A legal battle ensued. Rene had so many supporters that she was able to gather 55,000 signatures on a petition to allow Essiac Tea to be an officially recognized cancer treatment. The *Ontario Legislature* voted and she came up only three votes short of making it happen.

This led to a back and forth battle between her and the Canadian officials. They pressed for government trials, but she refused to give them the formula unless she got in writing that she wouldn't lose the rights to it because her loyalty was to the people and she wanted to keep treating them for free. They never provided any guarantees that she'd be keeping her formula rights, so she never gave it to them.

Rene also had visitors coming in from the *Memorial Sloan-Kettering Cancer Center* in New York City. They visited her regularly trying to get her to divulge the formula. She never complied.

Eventually the threat of imprisonment scared Rene into hiding and she closed her clinic doors in 1942.

Rene passed away in 1978 at the age of 90. Prior to her passing she had signed the rights to the Essiac Tea formula over to Dr. Charles Brusch, an old friend that she could trust, and former personal physician to John F. Kennedy. Brusch himself had used Essiac to cure his own cancer, and was indebted to Rene. She also signed the rights to the formula over to the *Respirin Corporation* of Toronto to test, manufacture and distribute Essiac Tea. The formula eventually became public after Rene gave it to her best friend, Mary McPherson. This certified true copy of Mary McPherson's two-page affidavit (scanned documents below) was provided by the *Commissioner of Affidavits* of the Town of Bracebridge, Ontario. Mary McPherson's affidavit is the only verifiable, legal evidence of Rene Caisse's Essiac formula. (Important note: the **root** of the sheep sorrel is an absolutely essential part of the formula):

Kenneth C. Dyer, Jr.

IN THE MATTER OF THE LATE RENE CAISSE

AND IN THE MATTER OF THE HERBAL REMEDY KNOWN AS "ESSIAC"

I, Mary McPherson of the Town of Bracebridge in the District Municipality of Muskoka, MAKE OATH AND SAY AS FOLLOWS:

1. I am presently 80 years of age. I have lived in Bracebridge area for most of my adult life.

2. I was well acquainted with the late Rene Caisse over the years from 1935 to 1978 during which time I assisted her.

3. I was fully aware that she made the decoction known as "Essiac" when she carried on her clinic at the Town of Bracebridge in the District Municipality of Muskoka, at 6 Dominion Street, Bracebridge, Ontario and at other locations in and about the Town of Bracebridge.

4. During the later years of the late Rene Caisse, I was responsible for the preparation of the herbal tea known as "Essiac", always under the supervision of the late Rene Caisse.

5. I confirm that the attached formula, set out in my own handwriting, and attached hereto as exhibit "A" to this my affidavit, <u>accurately</u> sets out the formula and the method of preparation which must be adhered to exactly as written for the herbal remedy known as "Essiac".

6. This affidavit is made in good faith and not for any improper purpose.

SWORN before me at the Town)

of Bracebridge in the District)　　_Mary McPherson_

Municipality of Muskoka)　　　　MARY McPHERSON

this 23 day of December, 1994)

_____
A Commissioner etc.

THIS IS CERTIFIED TO BE A TRUE COPY OF
THE

Janice M. Howden
JANICE M. HOWDEN, Deputy Clerk, for the Town of
Bracebridge, Commissioner for Affidavits, etc.

144

Essiac

6½ cups of burdock root (cut)
1 pound of sheep sorrel herb powdered
¼ pound of slippery elm bark powdered
1 ounce of turkish rhubarb root powdered

mix these ingredients thoroughly and store in glass jar in dark dry cupboard

Take a measuring cup use 1 ounce of herb mixture to 32 ounces of water depending on the amount you want to make.

I use 1 cup of mixture to 8×32 = 256 ounces of water Boil hard for 10 minutes (covered) then turn off heat but leave sitting on warm plate over night (covered In the morning heat steaming hot and let settle a few minutes then strain through fine strainer into hot sterilized bottles and set to cool store in dark cool cupboard. must be refrigerated when opened. When near the last when its thick pour in a large jar and sit in frig. overnight then pour off all you without sediment.

This recipe must be followed exactly as written
   I use a granite preserving kettle 10-12 qts)
   8 ounce measuring cup small funnel and fine strainer to fill bottles

The Heavy Handed Persecution of Royal Raymond Rife/The Bob Beck Protocol

Royal Raymond Rife was one of the world's greatest scientists who invented many things that are still in use today in electronics, optics, radiochemistry and biochemistry. In the 1920s he invented the world's first virus microscope. This invention was eventually featured on the front page of the *San Diego Union* newspaper on November 3rd, 1929. He had the enthusiastic endorsements of many doctors and researchers and was a highly respected individual.

At this point you should be asking yourself why you've never heard of this person. Like Nikola Tesla, one of the greatest geniuses in human history, this man has also been *systematically removed from all history books* and his legacy remains a **silent void**. Like I said before, anything that threatens the capitalist powers that be and their precious profits gets *suppressed*. Tesla had proven methods for creating *free energy*, and those methods would have wiped out the gas and oil industry, making it *obsolete* technology. Did you ever learn of Nikola Tesla in public school? Neither did I. Rife had a cure for all viral and bacterial diseases, and of course that would have wiped out most of the drug sales, therefore he too was omitted from history. Did you ever learn of him in school? Neither did I! Instead of going down in history as the geniuses that they were, they are *written out of history*. And that's the way things work when profits come first, anything that threatens their profits gets suppressed.

In 1933 Royal Raymond Rife, the father of "electromedicine", presented his very complex invention, the Universal Microscope, to the world. It utilized many quartz prisms and lenses, and with it Rife was able to magnify more than 60,000 times. Before this invention he was only able to magnify 2500 times. Those limitations frustrated Rife. Being the genius that he was he simply invented a new one. Unlike modern electron microscopes, which kill everything beneath them, with his new invention he observed the *living* cells growing and changing in form, making him the first human ever to see a live virus.

Rife quickly discovered that exposing bacteria and viruses to a certain *frequency* of radio waves would kill them almost instantly. This discovery led to him inventing a frequency instrument that created the exact frequencies needed to kill those bacteria and viruses. The principle is the same as a high pitched note that will break a wine glass. It does the same to all pathogens, parasites and viruses, basically increasing in frequency until they literally explode.

I have already discussed the concept of electromedicine in the chapter about MRSA, concerning the electromagnetic aspect of colloidal silver and how it kills the bacteria via electrical impulses and *not* via direct contact. Rife's machine behaves in precisely the same manner. Devices which mimic Rife's original are on the market known as "frequency generators" and can be found on various websites. The GB-4000 frequency machine is reportedly the best one out there and there is a website dedicated to it at: *TheGB4000.com*. The manufacturers aren't allowed to make medical claims, but medical advice regarding the machine can be obtained at the following website: *New-Cancer-Treatments.org*. Again, I'm not trying to advertise for any products in this book, I just want my readers to know their best options regarding their health. I'm simply passing on the information.

Another method of electromedicine is the Bob Beck "Blood Purifier" or the Hulda Clark "Zapper". I own the Bob Beck version. I simply attach the electrodes to my wrist at the main arteries and gently turn up the amperage to a comfortable level. The electricity is then transmitted to the blood effectively purifying it. The following is excerpted from my book *LOVE - EVOLVE - TRANSCEND: Building a Spiritual Culture on the Planet Earth*:

"Blood Electrification/Purification:

Gentle micro-currents (fifty to one hundred microamperes) of electricity are known to eliminate all viruses, parasites, fungi, bacteria and pathogens in blood and other liquids. The concept has been revealed in many revolutionary patents and research papers over the past one hundred plus years going back to 1897. Blood electrification takes two hours daily for about four weeks to get significant results.

Patents:

1897: Patent # 592735: —Apparatus for electrically treating liquids.
1972: Patent # 3692648: —Process For Oxygenating Blood and Apparatus for Carrying Out Same.
1973: Patent # 3753886: —Selective Destruction of Bacteria.
1976: Patent # 3994799: —Blood and tissue detoxification apparatus.
1986: Patent # 4616640: —Apparatus Birth control method and device employing electric forces.

1990: Patent # 5133932: —Blood processing apparatus.
1992: Patent # 5133352: —Method for treating herpes simplex.
1992: Patent # 5139684: —Electrically Conductive Methods and Systems for Treatment of Blood or other body fluids or synthetic Fluids.
1993: Patent # 5188738: —Alternating current supplied electrically conductive method & system for the treatment of blood or bodily fluids or synthetic fluids with electric forces.
2005: Patent # 6907294: —Apparatus and Methods for Facilitating Wound Healing.

Additionally, for areas of the body where the blood purification won't kill hazardous bacteria and viruses, such as in the lymph system, Dr. Beck devised a method of pulsing electromagnetic charges into those areas. His version utilizes a camera flasher rigged with a copper coil at the end which beams out pulses of electromagnetic energy into the area of the body that it's pressed up against, effectively purifying those areas. Again, from my book:

"High-intensity Pulsed Magnetic Fields:

Electromagnetic pulses sent to the lymph nodes, the spleen, kidneys & liver, help neutralize germinating, latent and incubating parasites of all types, helping to block re-infection. This speeds up the elimination of disease, restores the immune system, and supports detoxification. Bob Beck's device produces back EMF currents. You must have a high intensity, time varying, magnetic impulse for this to work. This process effectively reproduces the exact effect as mentioned in William A. Tiller's experiment in which the electromagnetic energy from the particles of colloidal silver in a beaker effectively kill the harmful bacteria in a separate beaker.

Patents:

1987: Patent # 4665898: —Malignancy treatment.
1987: Patent # 4665898: —Modification of the growth repair and maintenance behavior of living tissue and cells by a specific and selective change in electrical environment.
1987: Patent # 4654574: —Apparatus for reactively applying electrical energy pulses to a living body.
2004: Patent # 6675047: —Electromagnetic-field therapy method and device.

For more info on devices like this visit: *CancerTutor.com/bobbeck-bp* and/or read my first book *LOVE - EVOLVE - TRANSCEND: Building a Spiritual Culture on the Planet Earth.*

Now back to Royal Raymond Rife; In 1934 Dr. Milbank Johnson arranged formal clinical trials of Rife's Beam Ray device. Mr. Rife cured sixteen "terminal" cancer patients from *Pasadena County Hospital.* Every patient was 100% cured with absolutely no side effects!

What's even more interesting is that his treatments only lasted three minutes, after which the patient cleared their system for three days and then came back for more. Rife invested many years of study discovering the frequencies that specifically destroyed herpes, polio, spinal meningitis, tetanus, influenza, and numerous other diseases.

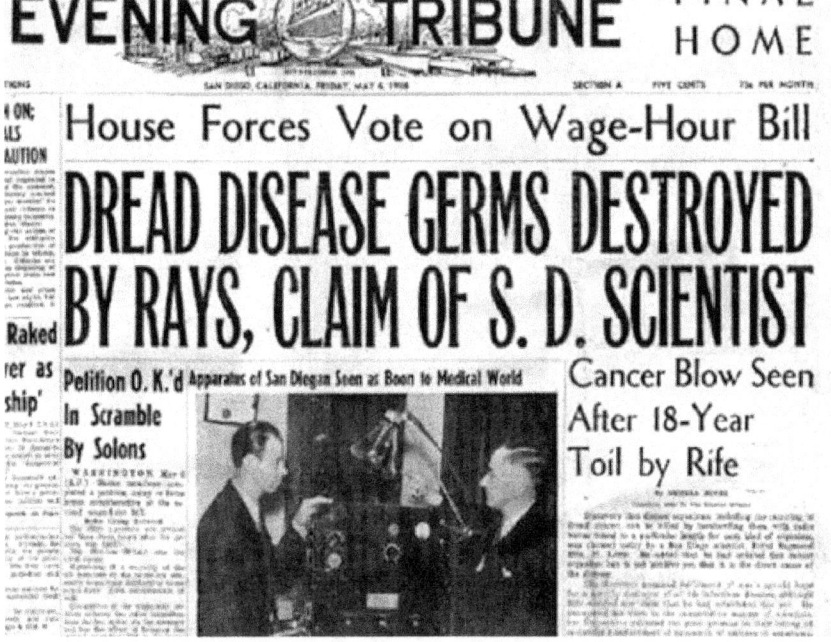

The Medical Mafia didn't like that very much. Morris Fishbein of the AMA, yes, the same Morris Fishbein from the Harry Hoxsey story above(!) offered to purchase Rife's machine from him. Of course, it was for the same reason as the Hoxsey case, he wanted to get rid of the Medical Mafia's competition. Like Hoxsey, Rife said **no way** and like Hoxsey, he was the victim of much heavy handed persecution. His lab was burned down, his microscope stolen, and some of the doctors who used Rife's equipment were raided. Two of those doctors were mysteriously found dead with *poison* in their system. The official word was "suicide". Yeah, right! The AMA also began revoking the licenses of doctors who used the Rife methods. People who were known to produce the equipment had it either confiscated or destroyed.

In 1944 Rife's friend, Dr. Milbank Johnson arranged a press conference to announce a cure for cancer to the world, Rife's Beam Ray device. The night before the announcement Johnson mysteriously turned up *dead*! It was eventually discovered that he *also* had poison in his system!

In the end Rife also had his 50 years worth of research records confiscated illegally, and none of the medical journals would print anything about his discovery. Rife was ruthlessly gagged and suppressed and his discoveries were lost in the huge pile of money and profits of the pharmaceutical industry and the *American Medical Association.*

You can obtain more information about Royal Raymond Rife by reading the book *The Cancer Cure That Worked* by Barry Lynes. There is a free e-book written by Carol Punt on how the body functions electrically entitled *Electricity for Health in the 21ˢᵗ Century* at the following URL:
www.naturalhealthproductions.com/pdf/electricityforhealthbooklet.pdf

The Persecution of Dr. Tullio Simoncini

Meet Dr. Simoncini, a Roman doctor with unorthodox, but effective methods of treating cancer. His book is entitled *Cancer is a Fungus* and because sodium bicarbonate ($NaHCO_3$) is one of the most powerful antifungal components in nature, that's what he uses to treat cancer. Yes, the main ingredient in baking soda!

Simoncini points to the similarities between cancerous cells and fungi like Candida, and in fact, claims that all cancer is an out of control fungal overgrowth (Candida) which occurs due to a *weakened immune system.* The list of similarities between cancer and fungi is quite extensive, and that it's a known fact that fungal infections *do cause cancer,* not to mention that they are very commonly correlated with leukemia, and all oncologists know that much.

> "Mycotoxins (fungal toxins) are genotoxic carcinogens, and exposure begins in utero and in mother's milk, continuing throughout life; these conditions favor the occurrence of disease."
>
> - *The American Cancer Society Textbook of Clinical Oncology*

Simoncini points out that all cancer infections are white in color, just like Candida, both cancer and fungi require *sugar* to live, they're both anaerobic (live without oxygen), both produce lactic acid and both are impacted by antifungal medicines.

Candida is normally kept under control by the immune

system, but when it becomes weakened the Candida can expand and build a "colony" just like cancer. Eventually it moves inside of the organs and the immune system responds by building a defensive barrier with its own cells, which is what a "tumor" is.

The Cancer Industry claims that the spreading of cancer to other parts of the body is caused by "malignant" cells escaping from their original location. Simoncini says that the spread of cancer is triggered by the Candida fungus, escaping from the original source.

Dr. Otto Warburg is the man who discovered cancer and who won a *Nobel Prize* for his work in 1931. In addition to his point that cancer feeds off of sugar, he emphasized two other main points in his book, which is entitled *Cancer: Its Cause and Its Cure*:

> "Cancer has only one prime cause, the replacement of normal oxygen respiration of body cells by an anaerobic cell respiration. Deprive a cell 35% of its oxygen for 48 hours and it may become cancerous."

and

> "No disease, including cancer, can exist in an alkaline environment."

Dr. Warburg emphasized that the root cause of cancer is oxygen deficiency, which induces an acidic state, and, of course, a lack of oxygen can cause fungal infection.

Dr. Warburg also discovered that because cancerous cells are anaerobic (do not require oxygen as normal cells do) and can *develop* from a lack of oxygen, they cannot survive in the *presence* of high levels of oxygen, as found in an alkaline state. He pointed out that if you want to prevent and cure cancer, the best way to go about that is to flood the system with oxygen and alkalinity as well as maintain a healthy diet *low in sugar.*

Concerning *sugar,* it not only induces an acidic state, it *feeds* cancer (and Candida). Cancer quite literally feeds off of glucose (sugar) as its main fuel source.

> "Cancer cells take in Glucose as a primary food; lactic acid is then excreted from the cancer cells into the blood. The blood carries the lactic acid to the liver, where it is converted back into glucose, which in turn feeds the cancer cells. This occurs in all known cancer cells. It has been so well documented for so long, that many years ago, serum glucose levels were used to monitor the progress of the disease. It was well established that as the disease progressed, serum glucose levels would rise.
>
> Knowing this, the wisdom of removing sugars and simple carbohydrates from the diet

becomes obvious. The ignorant use of glucose I.V.'s in cancer patients to administer medications also becomes painfully obvious. The object is to make it difficult for cancer cells to reproduce. Why fuel them with a primary requirement?

Likewise, cancer cells are unable to efficiently use protein or complex carbohydrates for food. But most importantly, the healthy cells of our body and immune system are able to use these as fuel, and for repair. It becomes imperative that we adapt the patient to a diet that includes protein and complex carbohydrates and eliminate the rest. Equally important, we must find treatment that not only attacks the cancer at a cellular level, but also feeds and improves the immune system at the same time."

- Dr. José Benavente, Director of Public Health, Ministry of Health, Valencia, Venezuela

What have I been saying about the low carbohydrate lifestyle in this book? I'll say it again: *"There is no dietary lifestyle that is healthier than the low carbohydrate lifestyle."* Like Dr. Jose' says above, not only does a low carb diet starve cancer cells of their main source of food (sugar, glucose), it gives them little else to live off of because cancer cells have a hard time using proteins as food. Additionally, the body can make great use of protein to enhance the immune system and to burn as fuel. The old myth that your body "needs" carbohydrates for fuel is just that, a *myth*. Proteins and fats burn just fine for fuel, which is why people on low carb diets lose weight so fast, they are quite literally burning their body fat as fuel. Leaving sugar and food that *turns into sugar* out of your diet is not only *protective against cancer and Candida*, it's simply one of the best things you can do for yourself. Period.

The best method of treating cancer is to create an *alkaline* state, and what's a better way to do that than with sodium bicarbonate? It's simply one of the best ways to combat acid and it floods *oxygen* into the body, which creates alkalinity and kills cancer. So why not make use of it? That's exactly what Dr. Simoncini did.

His method says that the best way to eliminate a tumor is to administer the sodium bicarbonate as close to it as possible, preferably right at the tumor. He administers it orally for cancer of the digestive tract, he uses enemas for rectal cancer, douches for uterine and vaginal cancer, injections for the lungs and brain, and inhalation for the upper respiratory. For internal organs he locates the arteries, for example the arteries in the liver, and pumps sodium bicarbonate in via a catheter. Depending on where the cancer is, he does his best to make sure that it comes into direct contact with the sodium bicarbonate. For skin cancers his treatment is a standard iodine tincture, a 7% solution.

According to Mark Sircus, Ac., OMD:

> "Dr. Simoncini routinely administers glucose with his IV treatments and this is the best indication for the use of either honey, maple syrup or blackstrap molasses especially for late stage cancer patients whose cells are starving."

The *reason* he uses sugary substances in conjunction with his sodium bicarbonate treatment is simple. He's tricking the cancer cells into opening up and making themselves vulnerable. He's pulling the "old switcheroo" because when the cancer cells know that sugar is on the way they are quick to open up for their favorite food source, but then all of a sudden here comes the sodium bicarbonate which floods the cancerous cells with oxygen and alkalinity, effectively killing them. I found an interesting article on *NaturalNews.com* that I'd like to share entitled *"Five year update on the guy who cured his stage IV prostate cancer with baking soda and molasses"*:

> "The guy is Vernon Johnston, and his story was first reported ... in 2009. That was around one year after being informed he was cancer-free from stage IV prostate cancer that had metastasized into the bone matter of his pelvic area in June of 2008.
>
> Now here it is, over five years later, and apparently Vernon's still going strong, according to his website reports, videos and announcements. The last known blog posting from Vernon was in August of 2013.
>
> That's five years and two months after being pronounced cancer-free at a Veterans Administration hospital.
>
> The mainstream medical standard for considering cancer cured is five years in remission or cancer-free. That self-imposed standard is rarely met with surgeries, radiation treatments and chemotherapy sessions. Many die from those treatments within five years!
>
> But after less than two weeks of intense bicarbonate of soda or baking soda (not baking powder) and blackstrap molasses consumption, he escaped not only cancer but toxic orthodox treatments.
>
> The baking soda/molasses combination caused a drastic pH alkaline spike that oxygenated his cancer cells to their demise. Since cancer cells thrive by fermenting sugar, the molasses was the bait that allowed baking soda's alkaline influence to enter and oxygenate them.
>
> He continued maintenance sessions every few months with two weeks of alkaline boosting using the same protocol of baking soda and molasses that he used to cure himself a few years ago..."
>
> **Full article is here**: *http://www.naturalnews.com/042525_stage_IV_prostate_cancer_baking_soda_treatment_five_year_update.html*

Dr. Simoncini points to many examples of brain tumors that have been spreading that have stopped dead in their tracks due to coming into contact with a 5% sodium bicarbonate solution. He reports that sodium bicarbonate has cured prostate cancer, intestinal cancer, stomach cancer, bladder cancer, breast cancer, spleen cancer, liver cancer, lung cancer, oropharyngeal cancer, peritoneal cancer, pancreatic cancer and others. When asked about his success rates he had the following to say:

> "My methods have cured people for 20 years. Many of my patients recovered completely from cancer, even in cases where official oncology had given up. If the fungi are sensitive to the sodium bicarbonate solutions and the tumor size is below 3 cm, the percentage will be around 90%, in terminal cases where the patient is in reasonably good condition it is 50%."

50% sure does beat chemotherapy's dismal 2.1%! All totaled Simoncini's success rate is about 80%, even better than Dr. Burzyinski's antineoplastons. Pretty amazing isn't it?

Dr. Simoncini is from Italy, but the same dark forces that control the *American Medical Association* also exercise the same power and control in most other countries. When he submitted his findings to the *Italian Department of Health* hoping that they would officially test it in government labs, his findings were completely ignored and he eventually lost his medical license, being completely disbarred from practice for using cures that aren't "approved" by them... *"for having administered sodium bicarbonate. Such practice has no scientific foundation, and it's not used in Italy"*. Never mind that it *works*, right!? That's beside the point. Let's just ignore that, ok? There are millions of people suffering and dying of cancer, but who cares, right? Let's take this amazing doctor's license away! And precisely *how* do they know there's "no scientific foundation" if they're totally and completely unwilling to test it in their labs? The true story is that they *know* it works, but they're not interested in that because it can't be patented and it's not *profitable*, that's the bottom line.

The good doctor was also the target of a major smear campaign via the mainstream media in Italy and repeatedly sued for "wrongful death" and in one case sentenced to three years in prison because he allegedly "caused" the deaths of some of his patients. Umm, with baking soda? How so? Chemotherapy is much better, right? Mainstream "doctors" kill millions with chemo, but when Dr. Simoncini loses a patient they blame it on the sodium bicarbonate! Ridiculous!

As an interesting side note, the ancient text of Ayurvedic medicine, humanity's oldest medicine system, entitled *Astanga Hrdayam* which is over one thousand years old, actually prescribes *"alkali of strong potency"* against *cancer.* It writes that these "should be used in diseases ... such as... *cancerous growth[s] which are very difficult to cure".* (Vol. I, *Sutra Sthana & Sarira Sthana*, page 346)

Dr. Simoncini's official website is at: CureNaturaliCancro.com

Sodium bicarbonate is a safe and natural substance, it's highly effective against cancer, and it's cheap. Hey, why the hell not? Would you rather use chemo? Be my guest.

Dr. Max Gerson: Poisoned by the Medical Mafia

Meet Dr. Max Gerson, a Jewish refugee of Nazi Germany who fled to New York City and started practicing his therapy of pure organic food, pancreatic enzymes and coffee enemas. He believed that cancer is caused by two main things; *deficiency* and *toxicity.* He stressed that lack of vital nutrients was at the core of cancer, as well as exposure to too many chemicals. He was correct, because all of those things damage the immune system. Back in the 1930s there were far less chemicals to worry about, and the rate of cancer was fairly low compared to that of today. Since the introduction of chemicals in our "food", our water, our air, etc the rates of cancer have exploded. Lack of proper nutrients is also proven to cause many diseases, not just cancer. If you don't feed your body what it requires it breaks down, and that's just common sense.

The *Gerson Therapy* developed as a result of Dr. Gerson's own personal health problems. He was having very serious migraine headaches and began experimenting on himself with his diet. Using a process of elimination he developed a diet that was an effective cure for those headaches. His conclusion was that foods such as creamy fish dishes, spicy sausages, alcohol, salt and fatty meats were causing those headaches.

The prime foundation of the Gerson Therapy is that initiating large amounts of vital nutrients from salt-free, fat-free, organic, vegetarian food, including 13 fresh organic vegetable and fruit juices daily. The idea is to flood the body's cells with vital nutrients, forcing out the toxins and allowing them to recover from that toxicity. And in order to help the liver process all of the toxins and get rid of them, part of Gerson's therapy was coffee enemas, which have taken a lot of ridicule, but are in fact, proven effective for that task.

I personally agree that flooding the body with nutrients is absolutely necessary in order to cure cancer naturally, and so is detox. The reason that so many herbal remedies are so effective for cancer is that they do three things; they provide nutrition, they assist in detox and they create an alkaline environment. And those three things combined strengthen the *immune system*. The vegetarian therapy obviously works, but I do not believe that eliminating proteins is healthy in the long run. If you have cancer, cutting out the red meats and fatty sausages for a while certainly wouldn't be a bad idea, but unless you're really sick and need to aggressively bombard yourself with nutrients as this diet recommends, I feel that getting adequate protein from animal sources is necessary for optimal health function. I know of a doctor named Nicholas Gonzalez who prescribes custom diets, including high protein, low carb "Atkins" type diets for his therapy, as well as an array of other diets, depending upon the patient's needs, which I'll address in the next section. Keep in mind what I pointed out earlier, and that is that *protein helps build a strong immune system*. A strong immune system is mandatory when treating cancer.

The *Gerson Therapy* works, and it works good, so I'm not knocking it, but it's my opinion that once the patient gets back on their feet, proper protein in the form of fish, chicken and limited red meats would be what's best. If you're dead set against meats you need to know that vegetarians are very typically extremely low in Vitamin B12, which can lead to hospitalization. Supplementing B12 is in your best interests, as the only source of B12 in nature is spirulina, which isn't commonly eaten as food.

In addition to an organic, vegetarian diet, pancreatic enzymes were also a very large part of Gerson's therapy. If the body has proper pancreatic enzymes the body can't develop cancer because they *dissolve the protective protein coating around malignant tissues*, making it impossible for them to grow and spread. More on that in the next section.

Eventually the Gerson Therapy was practiced on tuberculosis (TB) patients. In one study involving 450 terminal TB patients 446 of them recovered completely, which was considered a miracle because back then TB was considered to be "incurable". The Gerson Therapy was pretty well known in Europe because of that, and he put many TB clinics out of business as a result.

Eventually Gerson was begged by a woman who had incurable bile-duct cancer to treat her with his migraine and TB therapy. She knew it wasn't proven for cancer but was willing to try for lack of better options. She totally recovered and so did two of her friends who had cancers.

Shortly thereafter, Hitler started rounding up Jews and sending them to those fun camps, so Dr. Gerson got the hell out of there and went to New York City. When he arrived there he started promoting his "Gerson Therapy" to terminal cancer patients. In 1946, and with the support and presence of five of his cured cancer patients, Gerson testified in court that he had found the cure for cancer. On July 3rd, 1946 it was publicly announced on radio that the *Gerson Therapy* was a cure for cancer. During the same period he authored a book entitled *A Cancer Therapy: Results of Fifty Cases and the Cure of Advanced Cancer*, which is available on *Amazon.com*.

Of course, after he publicized his work as a cure for cancer, a smear campaign ensued. On March 8th, 1959, the good doctor mysteriously died. His daughter Charlotte recollects:

"My father, aged 78, was in perfectly good health when, from one day to the next, he felt awful. They tested his blood and found a high level of arsenic."

His daughter Charlotte opened the *Gerson Institute* in 1977 for the purpose of educating cancer patients about the Gerson Therapy. In response, the corrupt and immoral US government made the Gerson Therapy illegal, forcing Charlotte to move the clinic to Tijuana, Mexico. At this point you need to be asking yourself why anyone would want to make a vegetarian based *diet* in conjunction with pancreatic enzymes *illegal*. Clearly there is a bias here, and because it cures cancer it becomes totally obvious what that bias is. As a private citizen there's nothing they can do if you decide to use this therapy in the privacy of your own home, but if you open a clinic and start prescribing it you'd feel the consequences real fast. America is as corrupt as corrupt can get, and that's a simple fact.

The website of the *Gerson Institute* can be found at *Gerson.org*.

A Cancer Cure for Over 100 Years

Meet Dr. John Beard, a Scottish embryologist who invented the "trophoblast" theory sometime around the year 1900. Beard discovered some very interesting similarities between trophoblast cells and cancer cells which led him to write his book entitled *The Enzyme Theory of Cancer*, an overview of his theory and evidence.

My goal when writing this book was to keep things as simple as possible so that everyone can understand what's being said. I'm going to try to keep this simple, but it might seem a bit confusing at first. Please hang in there.

Dr. Beard noticed, first of all, that both trophoblast and cancer cells feature a protective coating around them; the trophoblast has a placenta and the cancer cell has a tumor. Both also have a source of nutrition; the trophoblast has an umbilical cord and the cancer cell has a new blood supply.

Trophoblast cells slow down activity at around the 8th week of pregnancy which coincides with the completion of the digestive system and the activation of the pancreas *in the fetus*. At this time, the hormone that is normally released from the trophoblast (human chorionic gonadotropin or "hCG") slows down as well. This hormone is the protective coating that is on trophoblast cells (and cancer cells!) to protect them *from the immune system*. This is highly interesting because only trophoblast cells and cancer cells produce this hormone. A positive urine test for hCG indicates one of two things; you're either a pregnant woman or you have cancer.

The reason that the hCG production slows down at the 8th week of pregnancy is, other than the completion of the fetus' digestive system and pancreas, because the fetus is now *producing enzymes* and those enzymes *break down the protective coating* on the trophoblast to begin the next stage of development. This is a key point. **Repeat**; the enzymes *break down* the protective coating.

Remember, this is a naturally occurring process during the course of a pregnancy, and cancer cells, as I've pointed out already, are very similar in that they have the same kind of protective coating. So by deductive reasoning it should make sense that *enzymes* would *also* break down the protective coating on the *cancer cells* too, yes? Are you following me? Good.

As an interesting side note, one of the rarest forms of cancer is cancer of the duodenum, the section of the intestines that is *highest* in pancreatic enzymes! Considering that the enzymes break down the barrier that protects cancer cells from the immune system, it makes all the sense in the world!

Unfortunately this cancer treatment never caught on, despite Dr. Beard publishing a book on his theory with evidence to back it up. It took another 60 years or so before anyone embraced the idea and tried to use it to treat cancer.

Meet Dr. William Donald Kelley, a Texas orthodontist, and the man who finally brought the pancreatic enzyme treatment of cancer to cancer patients. He discovered the enzyme therapy the hard way. He developed cancer at the age of 35. He had tumors in his pancreas, lungs, hip and liver. He thought he was a goner for sure, but his mother stepped in and demanded that he change his diet. She told him to eat nothing but raw foods; fruits, vegetables, nuts, grains and seeds. It took months but he began to feel better. Still battling cancer, he eventually developed some problems with his digestion, and so he decided to start taking enzymes. It was at this time that he also discovered the Dr. John Beard's long ignored book on pancreatic enzyme cancer therapy. After reading that book, he dramatically increased his dosage of enzymes, and amazingly he was eventually totally cured of cancer and never had any problems again.

Dr. Kelley went on to become a fantastic doctor who treated some 33,000 patients. Enzyme therapy takes a while to start working, consequently he did lose some patients who were too far along to be helped. But even with those issues, he still had an amazing cure rate of some 93%!

Dr. Kelley generally told his patients to modify their diets, eliminating pasteurized milk, peanuts, white flour, sugar, public treated water, and all processed foods. The Kelley diet plan varied depending upon the patient's needs; their cancer type and their metabolic type. Some patients would be prescribed a diet similar to the Gerson Therapy, strictly vegetarian and all raw foods, and some patients would be prescribed high protein, low carbohydrate "Atkins" type diets. Like Gerson, he also utilized coffee enemas for clearing out toxic buildup.

Curing so many people of cancer attracted the attention of the FDA, of course, and so they sent a young representative, a medical student by the name of Nicholas Gonzalez, to investigate and find flaws in his treatments. The goal was to prove Dr. Kelley wrong, to prove that his claims were untrue. Dr. Gonzalez showed up at Dr. Kelley's clinic in 1981 and was amazed to see patient after patient completely cured and doing just fine. Dr. Kelley opened up the files for Dr. Gonzalez, records of over 10,000 patients, and invited him to contact as many as he liked.

Despite the fact that the FDA's hitman wasn't able to prove Dr. Kelley wrong, he was eventually officially prohibited from treating anything but dental disease, and when he violated that order he was thrown in jail. (How dare you cure cancer! You're stealing our business!) He had also written a booklet entitled *One Answer to Cancer* that he was forbidden to circulate and publish! Yes, that's right. In the "land of the free" in the 1980s a man that was curing cancer over and over again was thrown in jail and forbidden to publish his book about it! God Bless America. The booklet that he was forbidden to publish is now available at the following URL: *www.drkelley.com/CANLIVER55.html*

Frustrated with the harassment of the Medical Mafia thugs, Dr. Kelley, like Gerson and Hoxsey, eventually moved his clinic to Mexico. He passed away in 2005, but he left us a book for our continuing education entitled *Cancer: Curing the Incurable Without Surgery, Chemotherapy or Radiation.*

The "hitman" that was sent by the FDA, Dr. Nicholas Gonzalez, was so impressed that he carried on Dr. Kelley's tradition and opened up a clinic in New York City where it remains (until he gets forced to Mexico like everyone else!). His website is at: *Dr-Gonzalez.com*. The book *Knockout: Interviews With Doctors Who Are Curing Cancer and How To Prevent Getting It In the First Place* by Suzanne Summers features an excellent interview with Dr. Gonzalez.

[Update for Second Edition: On July 21ˢᵗ, 2015 Dr. Gonzalez mysteriously died. The official word was a heart attack, but the doctor was in excellent health. He was 68. This happened after a string of fishy deaths, naturopathic doctors dropping like flies all of a sudden and for no apparent reason, all too convenient for the Medical Mafia and far too suspicious not to question.]

Cannabis Oil as the Cancer Cure: The Scientific Facts

Of all of the herbs in the world, *Cannabis Sativa* is by far the most demonized. Government propaganda against cannabis, hemp, marijuana, weed, or whatever you choose to call it, is monumental. But something that most people don't know about cannabis is that *it's one of the most useful plants in the history of the world, if not the most useful of them all.*

An article in *Popular Mechanics* in 1938 stated that there are more than 25,000 uses for cannabis/hemp. It can be used for rope, fabric, biodegradable industrial products, plastics, biomass fuels, replacement for wood products, paper, body care products, pet foods, detergents, art supplies, salad oil, and so on. "Hempcrete" is more energy efficient and stronger than standard concrete. One acre of hemp is equal to ten acres of trees and it makes more durable, longer lasting paper. The *Declaration of Independence* and the *Constitution of the USA* were drafted on hemp paper. George Washington and Thomas Jefferson grew hemp. Early laws in some American colonies *required* farmers to grow hemp, and they could be *jailed* for refusing to grow it! Henry Ford's first Model-T was made from plastic made out of *hemp fiber*, which was ten times stronger than steel. There is a video on *YouTube.com* where he swings a large ax against it and it fails to leave a mark! It shows no signs whatsoever of denting! Imagine trying to do that to your own car today! And just think, that technology has been blacklisted because certain people like to make money. What a crime. Additionally, that very same car was designed to run on ethyl alcohol extracted from hemp! *Hemp "gasoline"*! *Popular Mechanics* documented this fact in 1941 and various videos can be found on *YouTube.com*.

"The fuel of the future (ethyl alcohol) is going to come from fruit like that sumach out by the road, or from apples, weeds, sawdust -- almost anything. There is fuel in every bit of vegetable matter that can be fermented. There's enough alcohol in one year's yield of an acre of potatoes to drive the machinery necessary to cultivate the fields for a hundred years."

- Henry Ford

Additionally, the oil made from hemp seeds is quite sufficient to use in cars as an internal lubricant. As if this threat to the gas, oil and steel industries isn't enough, in the 1930s William Randolph Hearst and his paper manufacturing company supplied most of the paper as well as *newspapers* in the USA and were likely to lose billions of dollars in profits because of the hemp paper industry. During the same period *Dupont* had patented the process to make plastic out of oil and coal. As if that isn't enough to have a motive to remove hemp from the picture, from 1850 to 1937 medicinal cannabis was used as the prime medicine to treat over 100 separate illnesses or diseases in the *US Pharmacopoeia*. The *Smith Brothers, Parke Davis, Squibb, Lilly, Burroughs Wellcome* and other leading drug manufacturers marketed the product under the name of *"Extractum Cannabis"* and/or *"Extract of Hemp"*. But they had bigger plans, they had other, more profitable products in mind, and hemp was getting in the way. Clearly, cannabis was a conflict of interest for the drug cartels and numerous corporate swine institutions. Think about it; gas, oil and coal, lumber, plastic, steel, not to mention the medical industry and drug cartels...is it sinking in yet? Hemp was made illegal for the financial incentives of large corporations, not because it's "bad for you". If weed being "bad for you" was their reason, then why are cigarettes and alcohol still legal? Why is it ok to put cancer causing chemicals in our food, but an extremely useful and amazingly medicinal plant is against the law? Why would dangerous drugs be approved by the FDA, but cannabis is considered "dangerous"? Alcohol kills people all the time. Pot kills *nobody. Ever.* Clearly, something fishy is going on here, and I've already told you the reason.

Andrew Mellon was President Herbert Hoover's Secretary of Treasury at the time and he just happened to be the *largest investor in Dupont*. He appointed the husband of his niece (Harry J. Anslinger) to be in charge of the *Federal Bureau of Narcotics and Dangerous Drugs*. With everything set in motion, they had several behind closed door meetings with the corporate swine and conspired to make cannabis illegal. A massive propaganda campaign ensued. They gave it a slang name; "marijuana" to make it sound horrible and evil, the newspapers of Hearst ran stories on the "the devil's weed", films like *Reefer Madness* were produced, and a media heyday of massive propaganda was set in motion. (If you've never seen *Reefer Madness* I suggest you watch it. It's very clearly a propaganda film because it is so extremely *ridiculous* to watch. It has become a cult classic among pot smokers who sit and watch it as a form of entertainment.) Many corporate enterprises, the lumber industry, the gas and oil industry, and especially the drug industry stood to lose many billions of dollars if hemp wasn't very quickly removed from the picture. They all had financial incentives to destroy cannabis and make it illegal, and of course, they succeeded, because in a society where profits take top priority, the people with the money are the ones with the power and control.

Perhaps the most impressive use of cannabis is its medicinal value. It will do just about anything for you. It works as a pain killer, it relaxes the nerves, helps you sleep, relieves muscle aches and pains, assists with indigestion and stomach cramps, stimulates appetite, prevents people from becoming amputees by re-growing skin in gangrene infected areas, stops seizures, and much, much more. And, of course, it cures cancer.

Meet Rick Simpson, from Nova Scotia, Canada, perhaps the most well known advocate for the medicinal use of cannabis oil. His story starts in 1969 when his 22 year old cousin was diagnosed with cancer. He opted for surgery and chemotherapy. The "doctors" told him that they thought they'd "gotten it all" and he was ok for three years but then one day he suddenly collapsed in the presence of Rick. When he went to get checked out, as suspected, it was the cancer that had returned, which is all to common with cancer surgeries, they fail the vast majority of the time. This time they told him that he had three to six months to live, and within three months he was gone. This hurt Rick tremendously as they were very close.

About three years later, Rick was leaving work one day and he turned on the radio. He heard the announcers talking about the fact that THC, the main ingredient in cannabis, kills cancer cells. He said they were laughing so hard that he wasn't sure what to make of it. As time went on he never heard anything else about it, so he concluded that it was just "some type of hoax".

In 1997 Rick had a severe head injury at work, and wound up with "post concussion syndrome". His head rang 24 hours a day, which brought up his blood pressure, he had physical balance issues, and other associated problems. He said that he "went through the medical system and took their pills for five years and took every chemical they threw at me, but they did nothing but make me worse".

In 1998 he saw an episode of *The Nature of Things* produced by David Suzuki called *Reefer Madness II* and in that film he saw medical patients smoking marijuana and they were feeling better because of it. The first thing he did was go to a friend's house and get some pot and smoke it. He said it did more for him than anything the "doctors" were giving him. He repeatedly asked his "doctors" for a prescription for cannabis, but not a single one would comply. Eventually he asked one of them "what would you think if I made the essential oil of the plant and ingested it?" The "doctor" said that would be a much more medicinal way to use the substance, but that he still wouldn't give him a prescription. Despite the fact that the "doctor" knew that the only thing that was helping Rick was cannabis, and despite the fact that he knew that Rick would be charged with a crime if he was caught with it, he still refused all requests for a prescription.

Frustrated, Rick eventually started growing cannabis on his property, which is a large backwoods area out in a remote part of Nova Scotia, Canada. He then started producing his own cannabis oil and ingesting it. He said that it helped the ringing in his ears go away and he was able to sleep. He said nothing the "doctors" ever gave him helped him sleep. He also said that the arthritis in his knees disappeared. He lost about 25 pounds initially, which made him nervous because he was afraid that maybe the oil was hurting him, but he said that eventually his weight dropped to a certain level and just leveled off.

In 2002 he went to the "doctor" about what he thought was skin cancer and was diagnosed with basal cell carcinoma. He had two patches on his face and one on his chest. The one that he had next to his eye was a concern to his "doctors" because it was so close to the eye. They wanted to operate immediately and remove it. Rick got his surgery date and had the surgery. Afterwards he thought back to the time that he heard about THC killing cancer cells on the radio. At this point he was still skeptical but he decided to put it on his cancerous skin and see what happened. He simply dabbed some onto two band-aids and then put them on his two remaining patches. He left the band-aids on for four days, and when he took them off he was "shocked". He said it was all healed and there was just pink skin there. The cancerous patches that he had had for many years were gone, just that quick! He tried to tell people about it, but he was laughed at and called "crazy".

Eventually the cancerous patch that he had surgically removed came right back, as is common with cancer surgery. He simply put a band-aid on that spot for four days, took it off and it was healed. Ta-da! It's now 12 years later and those patches are still gone. He said that when he told the "doctor" how he had cured his cancer she "went ballistic" and made a scene in the waiting room in front of five or six other patients. It was on that day that Rick decided that he was no longer interested in "doctors" and decided to go it alone and just continue on with what he was doing, growing his own and producing his own oil.

Shortly after that incident, Rick's mother had really bad psoriasis on her feet so he took the oil over to her place and cured her psoriasis with it. Eventually he started giving treatments to various friends with skin conditions and "it was working on everything". He kept building and building, to friends of friends, and friends of their friends, etc.

Rick made several attempts to alert the government, but nobody would listen to him. He went to all of the political parties, he went to the *Cancer Society*, and he even went to the *United Nations*. But "nobody would lift a finger" he said.

In 2005 Rick put 1620 plants in his back yard and notified all authorities including the RCMP (*Royal Canadian Mounted Police*) of what he was doing, telling them why he was doing it and what it was for. He made a video tape and told them that it was for medicinal use for whoever needed it and he was not going to charge anything for it, it was all free. In other words, he was saving lives by helping people cure their cancers.

Not surprisingly, he was raided not too long after that and his plants were chopped down by the police. He admits now that he was naïve to think that they would actually take an interest in what he was doing, and be ok with it because it was saving people's lives. He believed in the system, as many people do, and did not realize the extent of the rampant corruption that runs our profit driven world. He said that while he was being raided one of the police told him that she believes everything he says about cannabis curing cancer. He stood there in disbelief and asked her "What are you doing? Where are your morals? Your friends are down there cutting down the cure for cancer for God sakes, now what's wrong with you people!?" The officer just went silent and said nothing further. He said that he had hundreds and hundreds of treatments worth of plants growing and he had lots of people waiting for their medicine, but the police showed no remorse as they chopped down his field.

In 2006 they did a second raid on Rick's property, and the local community was outraged. Rick had the support of the majority of the people in the area, including the *Royal Canadian Legion* and local police, and was considered a local hero because he had cured so many people of terminal cancers. Rick had called a town meeting to meet with the police, medical professionals, government representatives, etc. at the local *Royal Canadian Legion* branch, complete with patients that he had cured, etc. but the day before that was to happen the non-local police and non-local higher-ups from the legion came in and shut the local legion branch down. The *Royal Canadian Legion* suspended the entire management team of that local branch and refused to allow the building to be used for any meetings related to cannabis oil.

Rick is currently (at the time of writing) stuck in Europe, afraid to go home because his property was raided again, for the third time, while he was out of the country.

> "On November 25th, 2009, one day before I was crowned the Freedom Fighter of the Year at the Cannabis Cup in Amsterdam, I received word that I have been raided again by the RCMP. I contacted Tim Hunter at the Amherst detachment and asked if I was being charged. Of course, he refused to give me straight answer. All he would say was that the RCMP wanted to talk to me."

He's staying In Europe because if he's arrested when he comes home he'll be a third time offender and he knows they won't give him bail. If he's stuck in jail with no bail and no medicine he'll die. He says he's "not willing to commit suicide" by going back to Canada.

To date Rick has cured over 5000 patients. He still runs his website *PhoenixTears.ca* and has published some e-books which can be purchased there. *The Rick Simpson Story* is his story in his own words and *Cure for Cancer: The Rick Simpson Protocol* details his methods, from growing, to producing the oil, to dosages and other information. There is also a documentary about Rick entitled *Run From the Cure* on *YouTube.com* for your viewing pleasure. Enjoy.

The evidence that cannabis cures cancer is not confined to Rick's story. Far from it, as a matter of fact, Tommy Chong, of *Cheech and Chong* fame, was diagnosed with stage 1 prostate cancer in June of 2012. He knew about Rick Simpson, and so he used cannabis oil as a part of this therapy. Less than one year later he reported that he was "cancer-free". That was some great publicity for the fact that cannibinoids cure cancer.

> "After I came out with the news last June that a cancer doctor told me I had prostrate cancer and suggested a high frequency treatment that is not approved in America and could only be done in Mexico at the cost of $25,000, I immediately looked at alternatives. I contacted my nephew in Vancouver, who was about to become a doctor, and he suggested I meet with a Dr. McKinnon in Victoria, BC. That doctor changed my diet and put me on supplements, and within a year I brought my PSA numbers down drastically and eliminated the cancer threat. I also treated the condition with hemp oil (hash oil). With the diet, the supplements and the hash oil, plus a session with a world-renowned healer, Adam Dreamhealer, I'm cancer-free. That's right, I kicked cancer's ass! So the magic plant does cure cancer with the right diet and supplements. I'm due for another blood test, MRI, etc., but I feel the best I've felt in years. And now for a celebration joint of the finest Kush…"
>
> - Tommy Chong

This isn't scientific enough for you? Just an anecdote? "Where's the real evidence" you're thinking? Hmm. Well, ok then. Have a look at this link on the website of the *National Cancer Institute* entitled *"Cannabis and Cannabinoids–for health professionals (PDQ®)"*: http://www.cancer.gov/about-cancer/treatment/cam/hp/cannabis-pdq#section/all and take note of the link that says *"Antitumor Effects"*.

Still not good enough for you? Oh, ok. Well then. Here you go. Start with these:

Cannabinoids Cure Brain Cancer

A pilot clinical study of 9-tetrahydrocannabinol in patients with recurrent glioblastoma multiforme: http://www.nature.com/bjc/journal/v95/n2/abs/6603236a.html

Inhibition of glioma growth in vivo by selective activation of the CB(2) cannabinoid receptor: http://www.ncbi.nlm.nih.gov/pubmed/11479216

Neuroprotection by 9-Tetrahydrocannabinol, the Main Active Compound in Marijuana,

against Ouabain-Induced In Vivo Excitotoxicity:
http://www.jneurosci.org/content/21/17/6475.abstract

Antitumor Effects of Cannabidiol, a Nonpsychoactive Cannabinoid, on Human Glioma Cell Lines: *http://jpet.aspetjournals.org/content/308/3/838.abstract*

A Combined Preclinical Therapy of Cannabinoids and Temozolomide against Glioma: *http://mct.aacrjournals.org/content/10/1/90.abstract*

Cannabis extract makes brain tumors shrink, halts growth of blood vessels: *http://www.medicalnewstoday.com/releases/12088.php*

Cannabinoids Inhibit the Vascular Endothelial Growth Factor Pathway in Gliomas: *http://cancerres.aacrjournals.org/content/64/16/5617.full*

Triggering of the TRPV2 channel by cannabidiol sensitizes glioblastoma cells to cytotoxic chemotherapeutic agents: *http://carcin.oxfordjournals.org/cgi/content/full/34/1/48*

A Combined Preclinical Therapy of Cannabinoids and Temozolomide against Glioma: *http://mct.aacrjournals.org/cgi/content/full/10/1/90*

Cannabinoids inhibit the vascular endothelial growth factor pathway in gliomas: *http://www.ncbi.nlm.nih.gov/pubmed/15313899*

Cannabinoids Cure Mouth and Throat Cancer

Cannabinoids inhibit cellular respiration of human oral cancer cells: *http://www.ncbi.nlm.nih.gov/pubmed/20516734*

Cannabinoids Cure Breast Cancer

Pathways mediating the effects of cannabidiol on the reduction of breast cancer cell proliferation, invasion, and metastasis: *http://www.ncbi.nlm.nih.gov/pubmed/20859676*

Cannabidiol as a novel inhibitor of Id-1 gene expression in aggressive breast cancer cells: *http://www.ncbi.nlm.nih.gov/pubmed/18025276*

Crosstalk between chemokine receptor CXCR4 and cannabinoid receptor CB2 in modulating breast cancer growth and invasion: *http://www.ncbi.nlm.nih.gov/pubmed/21915267*

Anti-tumor activity of plant cannabinoids with emphasis on the effect of cannabidiol on human breast carcinoma: *http://jpet.aspetjournals.org/content/early/2006/05/25/jpet.106.105247.full.pdf+html*

Cannabinoids reduce ErbB2-driven breast cancer progression through Akt inhibition: *http://www.molecular-cancer.com/content/9/1/196*

Cannabinoids: a new hope for breast cancer therapy?: *http://www.ncbi.nlm.nih.gov/pubmed/22776349*

The endogenous cannabinoid anandamide inhibits human breast cancer cell proliferation: *http://www.pnas.org/content/95/14/8375.full.pdf+html*

Drugging for "Health": Why the Paradigm Must Change

9-Tetrahydrocannabinol Inhibits Cell Cycle Progression in Human Breast Cancer Cells through Cdc2 Regulation: *http://cancerres.aacrjournals.org/content/66/13/6615.abstract*

Synthetic cannabinoid receptor agonists inhibit tumor growth and metastasis of breast cancer: *http://mct.aacrjournals.org/content/8/11/3117.full*

Betulinic Acid Targets YY1 and ErbB2 through Cannabinoid Receptor-Dependent Disruption of MicroRNA-27a:ZBTB10 in Breast Cancer: *http://mct.aacrjournals.org/cgi/content/full/11/7/1421*

Cannabinoids Cure Lung Cancer

Cannabidiol inhibits lung cancer cell invasion and metastasis via intercellular adhesion molecule-1: *http://www.ncbi.nlm.nih.gov/pubmed/22198381?dopt=Abstract*

Cannabinoid receptors, CB1 and CB2, as novel targets for inhibition of non-small cell lung cancer growth and metastasis: *http://www.ncbi.nlm.nih.gov/pubmed/21097714?dopt=Abstract*

9-Tetrahydrocannabinol inhibits epithelial growth factor-induced lung cancer cell migration in vitro as well as its growth and metastasis in vivo: *http://www.nature.com/onc/journal/v27/n3/abs/1210641a.html*

Cannabinoids Cure Pancreatic Cancers

Cannabinoids Induce Apoptosis of Pancreatic Tumor Cells via Endoplasmic Reticulum Stress–Related Genes: *http://cancerres.aacrjournals.org/content/66/13/6748.abstract*

Cannabinoids Cure Prostate Cancer

Anti-proliferative and apoptotic effects of anandamide in human prostatic cancer cell lines: implication of epidermal growth factor receptor down-regulation and ceramide production: *http://www.ncbi.nlm.nih.gov/pubmed/12746841?dopt=Abstract*

The role of cannabinoids in prostate cancer: Basic science perspective and potential clinical applications: *http://www.ncbi.nlm.nih.gov/pmc/articles/PMC3339795/tool=pubmed*

Non-THC cannabinoids inhibit prostate carcinoma growth in vitro and in vivo: pro-apoptotic effects and underlying mechanisms: *http://www.ncbi.nlm.nih.gov/pubmed/22594963*

Cannabinoids Cure Colorectal Cancer

Chemopreventive effect of the non-psychotropic phytocannabinoid cannabidiol on experimental colon cancer: *http://www.ncbi.nlm.nih.gov/pubmed/22231745*

Cannabinoids Cure Colon Cancer

The Cannabinoid WIN 55,212-2 Decreases Specificity Protein Transcription Factors and the Oncogenic Cap Protein eIF4E in Colon Cancer Cells: *http://mct.aacrjournals.org/content/12/11/2483.full*

Induction of Apoptosis by Cannabinoids in Prostate and Colon Cancer Cells Is
Phosphatase Dependent: *http://ar.iiarjournals.org/cgi/content/full/31/11/3799*

Cannabinoid Receptor Activation Induces Apoptosis through Tumor Necrosis Factor
{alpha}-Mediated Ceramide De novo Synthesis in Colon Cancer Cells:
http://clincancerres.aacrjournals.org/cgi/content/full/14/23/7691

Cannabinoids Cure Blood Cancer (Leukemia)

Targeting CB2 cannabinoid receptors as a novel therapy to treat malignant lymphoblastic
disease: *http://www.ncbi.nlm.nih.gov/pubmed/12091357*

Delta 9-tetrahydrocannabinol-induced apoptosis in Jurkat leukemia T cells is regulated by
translocation of Bad to mitochondria.: *http://www.ncbi.nlm.nih.gov/pubmed/16908594*

Expression of cannabinoid receptors type 1 and type 2 in non-Hodgkin lymphoma:
Growth inhibition by receptor activation:
http://onlinelibrary.wiley.com/doi/10.1002/ijc.23584/abstract

Cannabinoid Receptor-Mediated Apoptosis Induced by R(+)-Methanandamide and
Win55,212-2 Is Associated with Ceramide Accumulation and p38 Activation in Mantle
Cell Lymphoma: *http://molpharm.aspetjournals.org/content/70/5/1612.abstract*

Cannabinoids Cure Skin Cancer

Inhibition of skin tumor growth and angiogenesis in vivo by activation of cannabinoid
receptors: *http://www.ncbi.nlm.nih.gov/pubmed/12511587*

Cannabinoids Cure Liver Cancer

Anti-tumoral action of cannabinoids on hepatocellular carcinoma: role of AMPK-
dependent activation of autophagy: *http://www.ncbi.nlm.nih.gov/pubmed/21475304*

Cannabinoids Cure Biliary Tract Cancer

The dual effects of delta(9)-tetrahydrocannabinol on cholangiocarcinoma cells: anti-
invasion activity at low concentration and apoptosis induction at high concentration:
http://www.ncbi.nlm.nih.gov/pubmed/19916793

Cannabinoids Cure Cancer in General

Inhibition of tumor angiogenesis by cannabinoids:
http://www.ncbi.nlm.nih.gov/pubmed/12514108

Potentiation of Cannabinoid-Induced Cytotoxicity in Mantle Cell Lymphoma through
Modulation of Ceramide Metabolism:
http://mcr.aacrjournals.org/cgi/content/full/7/7/1086

When you're done letting those studies sink in, go to
Scholar.Google.com and type the following into their search box:
"cannabinoids cancer". I just did the search myself and it yields

21,500 results. I'd say that the evidence is clear that "the devil's weed" cures cancer. That secret isn't so secret anymore.

In 1974 researchers at the *Medical College of Virginia*, who were funded by the *National Institute of Health*, were doing a study trying to prove that marijuana damages the immune system. They didn't find their proof, but they did find that THC slowed down the tumors of three different types of cancer in mice. Instead of getting happy and excited the government immediately shut down that study.

And get a load of this story from *LeafScience.com* entitled *"Drug Maker Will Soon Hold Patent On THC, CBD As Cancer Cures"*:

"GW Pharmaceuticals announced Wednesday that it has been issued a Notice of Allowance from the U.S. Patent Office for a patent application involving the use of THC and CBD, the two main chemicals in marijuana, for treating gliomas.

Once a patent application is deemed a genuine invention, the Patent Office sends a Notice of Allowance that outlines the fees involved with final approval.

Specifically, the company provides this description of the patent:

"The subject patent specifically covers a method for treating glioma in a human using a combination of cannabidiol (CBD) and tetrahydrocannabinol (THC) wherein the cannabinoids are in a ratio of from 1:1 to 1:20 (THC:CBD) with the intent to reduce cell viability, inhibit cell growth or reduce tumor volume."

Filed in 2009, GW's patent application lists Otsuka Pharmaceutical as a collaborator and initially claimed the invention of the "use of a combination of cannabinoids in the manufacture of a medicament for use in the treatment of cancer."

However, it's likely that the application was revised since then to be more specific in its claims, including the ratio of THC to CBD used and the type of cancer treated.

Indeed, the use of cannabis and cannabis-derived chemicals to fight a wide range of cancers has long been suggested by pre-clinical research as well as anecdotal reports.

On the other hand, the first clinical trial to investigate these cancer treatments only began last month, launched by GW Pharmaceuticals for their cannabis drug Sativex.

The trial investigates Sativex in combination with the standard chemotherapy drug temozolomide, and involves 20 patients with recurrent glioblastoma multiforme (GBM), an aggressive and rare form of brain cancer.

GW Pharmaceuticals also announced in November that it had begun human trials of a CBD-rich cannabis drug for the treatment of pediatric epilepsy."

Full article is here: *http://www.leafscience.com/2013/12/13/drug-maker-will-soon-hold-patent-thc-cbd-cancer-cures/*

As you can see, drug companies know what's up, and they're trying

to capitalize on it. But it won't work. Isolating the two chemicals in weed that kill cancer won't work nearly as well, because there are numerous other chemicals in herbs that work together synergistically. When you isolate single chemicals to make drugs, the synergistic properties of the plant are destroyed, and drugs that are made in that fashion never, *ever* work as good as the original herb. But the original herb can't be patented, you see, that's why they try to isolate only certain parts of the plant. But even so, chemotherapy is too lucrative to consider releasing something like this. It would hurt their profits more than help them make money. The likely scenario is that they'll just sit on the patent and let it collect dust. But they *did* get their patent. *"Phytocannabinoids in the treatment of cancer"* US Patent # US 20130059018:
http://www.google.com/patents/US20130059018

Also, on Oct. 7th, 2003 the US Government as represented by the *Department of Health and Human Services* was granted US Patent # 6630507 on any and all uses of *"Cannabinoids as antioxidants and neuroprotectants"*: http//goo.gl/tdwtb

When it comes to cannabis, we've all been had. When it comes to *cancer*, we've all been had. **Clearly, cancer is curable**. And clearly, the dark powers that run our so-called "medical" system need to be destroyed so that *honest* practices can be put into place making it possible for proven natural methods to be recognized and used to their fullest potential, instead of *systemically and intentionally ignored and suppressed* by a bunch of corporate swine who care about nothing but money. Clearly, the paradigm must change!

> "Millions of people have died horrible deaths and in many cases, families exhausted their savings on dangerous, toxic and expensive drug. Now we are just beginning to realize that while marijuana has never killed anyone, marijuana prohibition has killed millions."
>
> - Raymond Cushing

Like the Energizer Bunny,
the List of Cancer Cures Continues...

You didn't think I was done yet did you? I'll be honest with you, I thought that I was almost done writing this book. I thought that the research that I'd done previously concerning cancer was complete enough. But when I started doing additional research for this book, what I found *dumbfounded* me. I have discovered that protocols for cancer that are effective, protocols that *work*, are all over the place! There is an abundance of them! If I've gained anything through writing this book, it's knowledge of cancer and how to treat it, and I am very happy to share that information with you, my readers, *especially if you have cancer*! But again, please do consult your primary care provider, preferably a naturopathic doctor, before starting any new programs! Especially if you have cancer! I'm providing you with this information for your education only!

Something that I've noticed about many of these protocols is that they have much in common. Most of them share three basic rules and those are **1)** boosting the immune system **2)** detoxing the body and the blood and **3)** dietary changes. In a nutshell; clearing out the bad stuff, and building up the good stuff. Basic common sense, as opposed to what mainstream "doctors" do; load you up with *toxic shit* (chemotherapy, radiation) which *destroys the immune system and poisons your body*, pretty much guaranteeing your imminent death. Generally, most cancers can be reversed by detoxing the system and boosting immunity. Some of the protocols that I've listed so far make no mention of those things, they simply show how to kill cancer cells, but if you have cancer, trust me, you need to detox and you need to adjust your diet. That goes without saying. If you're eating at McDonalds you can just forget it, if you're doing chemotherapy or radiation you can just forget it. You'll die! Poison won't magically make you healthy, it simply doesn't work that way, sorry. If you don't want to die, *flush your system and eat a nutritious diet.* Cleanse and detox! Very important! How? By using organic foods *as medicine* and taking herbs and other supplements.

There is a specific order in which you must do your detox. Think of it this way; why do a blood cleanse if your liver is still full of toxins? Your liver will simply flood the blood stream with toxins and then you will than have done a blood cleanse for nothing. You need to cleanse the liver first. Generally, the blood cleansing is the very last thing on the list. And that's just one example of why you must detox in *proper order.* This is the order suggested by most natural health practitioners:

1) Colon Cleanse
2) Parasite Cleanse
3) Kidney Cleanse
4) Liver/Gall Bladder Cleanse
5) Blood Cleanse

Right now I'd like to share lists of the best herbs for each phase. Unless you're an herbalist who knows how to effectively make your own blend, I recommend that you either visit your local health food store for good cleanse formulas, or shop online. You'll want to make sure you get a good quality product that uses organic herbs. Shop around a bit. Generally, the cheaper it is, the *cheaper it is*! Don't penny pinch on your detox! If it was me personally, I'd order bulk herbs from a quality vender that sells only the best organic herbs and then make my own tinctures. That's by far the best way to guarantee quality. Tinctures are easy to make and you can simply Google "how to make an herbal tincture" to learn how.

Phase 1 - Herbs that detox the colon (cathartics):

- Alfalfa
- Aloe Vera
- Boswellia
- Buckthorn Bark
- Chamomile
- Fennel Seed
- Fenugreek
- Flax Seed
- Grapefruit Pectin
- Gentian
- Goldenseal
- Guar Gum
- Horehound
- Licorice Root
- Marshmallow
- Papaya Fruit
- Peppermint
- Psyllium
- Raspberry
- Rhubarb
- Sangre de drago
- Slippery Elm

- Uva Ursi
- **Note: Coffee Enemas are also highly recommended**

Phase 2 - Herbs that remove parasites (parasiticides):

- Artemisia
- Barberry
- Betel Nut
- Black Walnut Hulls
- Bromelain
- Cascara Sagrada
- Chaparral
- Clove Bud
- Echinacea
- Garlic
- Gentian
- Goldenseal
- Pau D'Arco
- Prickly Ash
- Sage
- Tansy
- Thyme
- Wormwood
- **Note: Parasite cleansing is generally far *more effective when fasting.* I've read reports that the best synergistic blend for parasites is <u>Black Walnut Hulls, Wormwood and Cloves.</u>**

Phase 3 - Herbs that cleanse the kidneys (diuretics):

- Agrimony
- Burdock Root
- Cardamom
- Celery
- Chanca Piedra
- Coptis
- Corn Silk
- Couch Grass
- Dandelion
- Echinacea
- Goldenrod
- Goldenseal
- Gravel Root
- Horsetail
- Hydrangea Root
- Marshmallow Root
- Parsley
- Scutellaria
- Stinging Nettle
- Uva Ursi

Phase 4 - Herbs that cleanse the liver and gallbladder (hepatics):

- Artichoke

- Barberry
- Burdock Root
- Chanca Piedra
- Chicory
- Dandelion
- Fenugreek
- Maitake
- Milk Thistle
- Peppermint
- Reishi
- Schisandra
- Tumeric
- Yellow Dock

Step 5 - Herbs that cleanse the blood (alteratives):

- Alfalfa
- Angelica
- Barberry
- Burdock Root
- Butcher's Broom
- Cayenne
- Chaparral
- Chickweed
- Comfrey
- Dandelion
- Devil's Claw
- Echinacea
- Gingko
- Ginseng
- Goldenseal Root
- Green Tea
- Hawthorn
- Horse Chestnut
- Nettles
- Olive Leaf
- Prickly Ash
- Pygeum
- Quercitan
- Red Clover
- Saw Palmetto
- Uva Ursi
- Witch Hazel
- Yellow Dock

The idea is to **detox and fortify**. Get rid of the toxins and fortify the nutrients. **Detox and fortify**. Adding in more toxins (chemotherapy) and destroying the immune system simply isn't an option. You need to *get rid of* the toxins, and *build* the immune system! Again, simple common sense, the direct opposite of what "doctors" do!

You've already seen that the Gerson and Kelley/Gonzalez therapies involve dietary changes. They both encourage all organic foods, and depending on your body type and metabolism type you may or may not want to discontinue eating meats. Gerson stipulates no meats, period, while Kelley/Gonzalez modify diets accordingly for every individual patient. Some of them get vegetarian diets, some of them don't, it just depends. Concerning other dietary protocols, there are many, and again, the common thread is cleansing and building immunity. I've heard it called "overdosing on nutrition", which sounds good to me. Instead of overdosing on poison (chemotherapy) while mainstream medicine laughs all the way to the bank as you plan your funeral arrangements, simply overdose on nutrition instead and see how much better you'll be doing!

The Budwig Diet

Dr. Johanna Budwig, a German biochemist and seven time *Nobel Prize* nominee was an expert on essential fatty acids (EFAs) and an employee of the German government during the 1950s. She observed that the (cooking) oils commonly used by society are mostly all *chemically altered* by the companies who sell them because it gives them a longer shelf life. She referred to these chemically altered fats as "psuedo-fats". Dr. Budwig observed that these pseudo-fats destroy the electrical fields of the cells, effectively causing the oxidase ferments to be destroyed by heating or boiling. To put it another way, they caused the cells to be lacking in oxygen and lower in electrical voltage, effectively causing the cells to be cancer-prone. If you remember from the section on Dr. Simoncini, cancer cells can't live in the presence of oxygen, but they thrive in a low oxygen environment. The oil's damage to the cells creates a perfect environment for cancers to grow.

Upon examination of patients bloodwork, Dr. Budwig discovered that the blood of cancer patients was always deficient in essential fatty acids (lipids), while at the same time the blood of healthy patients was always the exact opposite of that. When looking at cancer patient's blood, instead of seeing the rich, red, oxygenated hemoglobin that she saw in healthy patients, she saw a greenish-yellow substance instead. Not good! She hypothesized that if she replaced those missing fats perhaps it would assist in the healing of the patient, and sure enough it did. She found that when those fats were replaced, the cancerous tumors started shrinking. This is the part where many people shake their heads in disbelief; in order to replace those fats she fed her patients a combination of *cottage cheese* and *flaxseed oil*! Flaxseed oil is rich in electrons and EFAs (which helps to repair the electrical charge of the cells) and cottage cheese is high in sulfur-rich proteins (which helps to give the cells their much needed EFAs). Both serve to *bind oxygen* (which destroys cancer) and reinvigorate the cells destroyed by the chemically altered psuedo-fats. As incredible as it sounds, this therapy shrinks cancerous tumors. She had much success with her work, cured many people, and of course, she was persecuted for it. Eventually her funding was cut off by the German government, she was fired from her job and she was also prevented from publishing her findings.

> "I have the answer to cancer, but American doctors won't listen. They come here and observe my methods and are impressed. Then they want want to make a special deal so they can take it home with them and make a lot of money. I won't do it, so I'm blackballed in every country."
>
> - Dr. Johanna Budwig

A modern American doctor by the name of Bill Henderson has carried on the Budwig tradition. His main focus is a very strict diet plan based on the Budwig protocol, he has worked with thousands of patients and has a very high success rate. His book *Beating Cancer Gently* can be purchased at his website: *Beating-Cancer-Gently.com*. Further research on the Budwig therapy can be conducted at *BudwigCenter.com*.

Johanna Brandt's "Grape Cure"

Johanna Brandt of South Africa cured herself of stomach cancer in the 1920s using what she called *The Grape Cure*. The Brandt protocol involves a strict diet of grapes, grape mush, grape juice and water. The protocol involves 12 hours of fasting (water only) per day followed by 12 hours of grape consumption and supplement intake. This is done for six weeks at a time.

You'll need organic grapes, obviously, and purple concord grapes specifically, as they seem to be the highest quality. During the fasting period you're encouraged to drink lots of water, a minimum of half a gallon during fasting and half a gallon during the grape consumption period. During the grape consumption period you're supposed to eat at least a half gallon of grape mush, including the seeds, which you prepare in a food processor. Spread the consumption out to at least 8 eating periods over the course of the 12 hours. Grapes, grapes, and more grapes. You will also be consuming several supplements; grape seed extract, grape skin extract, quercitan, Vitamin C, cayenne pepper and niacin.

Crazy is it? Well, yes, it certainly sounds crazy if you don't understand why it works. It sounds totally unbelievable I know, almost as unbelievable as cottage cheese and flaxseed oil! But the fact of the matter is that grapes contain an *army* of powerful cancer fighting substances including ellagic acid, lycopene, OPCs, selenium, catechin, quercitan, gallic acid and Vitamin B17 (amygdalin). But the most prevalent ingredient in grapes that does most of the cancer fighting is called **resveratrol**. Resveratrol is a bioflavonoid that is produced in the skin of grapes for the purpose of protecting the grapes from pathogens. It has very powerful *antifungal* and *antibacterial* properties. When we think back to the section that I wrote about Dr. Simoncini and his baking soda cure, we'll remember that there is a long list of similarities between cancer and fungus. Resveratrol kills candida fungus quite effectively, and because of that, of course it kills cancer cells too.

Resveratrol induces apoptosis (cellular suicide or cell self-destruction) of cancer cells and numerous scientific studies back up that fact. Again, I'd like to direct you to *Scholar.Google.com*. Type in "resveratrol cancer" and have a look. When I did the search I got **64,800** results. Resveratrol is also available as a supplement, in powders and capsules. Taking resveratrol along with quercitan and bromelain is a very powerful synergistic combination.

<u>Other Nutrition Based Cancer Fighters</u>

As you've seen, nutrition is the most powerful weapon that there is against cancer. Common herbs, organic fruits and vegetables, healthy fats like cottage cheese and flaxseed oil, baking soda, pancreatic digestive enzymes, and so forth and so on, all have very powerful anticancer benefits, and when you take all of those dietary therapies and *combine them* all with other anticancer supplements you have a mighty arsenal that most likely cannot be defeated. But you can't allow yourself to be *contaminated* with more toxins! As someone with cancer you're already toxic, the idea is to detox, *not* add in more toxins, therefore chemotherapy is out of the question and so is radiation! *They don't work! They kill!* I'm not trying to sound like a broken record, repeating myself over and over again, but I really can't emphasize that enough, that point needs to be hammered in. If you want to live you won't do chemotherapy or radiation, you'll embrace real treatments that *work* instead. Gee, what a concept.

As someone with cancer you'll not only require a detox and a healthy diet plan, you'll require numerous supplements. The idea is to cover all of your bases. If you have, for example, a deficiency in magnesium, or anything else for that matter, that will just make your battle with cancer that much more more difficult. You need to cover all of your vitamins, minerals, fats, proteins and amino acids and make sure you drink plenty of *purified water*, at least one gallon per day.

Distilled water is not recommended because even though it is pure, it's *dead*. It doesn't contain necessary nutrients. Distilled water is also very **acidic**. Your best bet for drinking water is a high quality water filter for your home. If that's not possible bottled *alkaline* water from your local health food store is your next best bet. I personally purchase purified drinking water water from my local grocery store, and then I pump **ozone** into it for further purification. If you drink the water soon after pumping ozone into it, your body will receive the same purification benefits as the water not to mention an *oxygen boost*, which I've already shown is very good for killing cancerous cells. It's a very powerful way to cleanse the system. I personally chug down three one quart jugs of ozonated water daily, plus I drink lots of iced tea as well, which is very high in antioxidants, also good for combating cancerous cells. Ozone pumps are quite inexpensive, simply go to *Google.com* and do a search. I believe I paid about $89.00 for mine including shipping. I've had it for over five years now and it still works like a champ.

I'd like to list off some additional weapons for your cancer fighting arsenal right now. Many of these products have several ingredients. Some are herbal formulas, some are multi-vitamin/mineral supplements with other things added in, and some are just powerful cancer fighters all by themselves. Once again I'd like to mention that I'm not looking to advertise for anyone in this book, that's not the idea behind listing various products here, the idea is to be *complete* and make sure that you know what your real options are. There are many! I just wouldn't feel right if I left some of these things out just because they're commercial products. They're powerful cancer fighters and I want my readers to know about them. So here they are:

Cellect: *Cellect* powder is a *nutritional powerhouse*. It's commonly used in conjunction with the Budwig diet, known as the "Cellect-Budwig Diet", and it's jam packed with various vitamins, minerals (including 74 trace minerals) and amino acids. It also has some anticancer agents added in as well, shark cartilage being the main one (for the science behind shark cartilage as a cancer treatment go to *Scholar.Google.com* and type in "shark cartilage cancer"). It's results with cancer are outstanding. *Cellect* was invented by Fred Eichhorn, a biochemist who had "terminal" pacreatic cancer in 1976. He still lives today, and is the President of the *National Cancer Research Foundation* (*NCRF.org*). You can read up on his amazing supplement and protocol, as well as order the product at *Cellect.org*.

LifeOne: LifeOne is another nutritional powerhouse, this one containing mainly herbal ingredients. It's a liquid tincture in a liposomal base, which preserves the ingredients and provides for better absorption. *LifeOne* and its ingredients have all been through lots of testing, and it showed to be effective against *all* cancer lines tested. It has shown to cure cancer in animals and in human patient treatments involving many cancers; hepatic, renal, lung, glioblastoma multiforma, invasive ductal cell carcinoma, oligodendroglioma, bladder, colon, pancreatic, melanoma, sarcomas, brain tumors and small cell cancers. The ingredients in *LifeOne* are some of the most powerful anticancer agents in nature. They include:

> **Chrysin**: A flavonoid from the Passion Flower that has antioxidant effects, inhibits 6 of the 7 procancer events, enhances Tumor Necrosis Factor (TNF) cytotoxicity to cancer cells.

> **Coriolus Versicolor**: A Chinese herbal mushroom with anticancer effects, potently stimulates the immune system, inhibits the invasion of cancer cells (metastasis and local proliferation), inhibits 4 of the 7 procancer events.

> **Diindolymethane (DIM)**: DIM is a phytochemical from cruciferous vegetables (broccoli, Brussels sprouts, cabbage), inhibits adhesion, motility, and invasiveness of cancer cells, inhibits 5 of the 7 procancer events.

> **Resveratrol**: Non-flavonoid phenolic compound found in grapes, inhibits 6 of the 7 procancer events.

> **Turmeric Extract (Curcumin)**: Acts as a potent antioxidant, inhibits cancer cell proliferation in vitro, inhibits metastasis in vivo, inhibits 5 of the 7 procancer events.

> **Quercetin**: A flavonoid that induces cell apoptosis, inhibits 6 of the 7 procancer events.

> **Green Tea Extract**: A flavonoid containing epigallocatechin gallate (EGCG), the primary anticancer agent, in-vitro and in-vivo anticancer activity, inhibits 6 of 7 procancer events.

> **L-Selenium Methionine**: The organic form of selenium, which is better utilized by the body, inhibits 6 of the 7 procancer events, in-vitro and in-vivo studies show anticancer effects, strong immune stimulator.

> "For a comparison with the LifeOne Formula, TAXOL, the number one chemotherapy ingredient in the world, is derived from a single natural ingredient that comes from the bark of the Pacific Yew tree which is then chemically reproduced in pharmaceutical laboratories and it no longer has anything natural about it. The LifeOne Formula contains more than 8 active natural ingredients obtained from around the world, all of which work synergistically in a liposomal delivery system to produce an unequaled attack against cancer. The complete story and history of the LifeOne Formula can be found at: *HealthPro.com.dm*."

> - Dr. Jose' Benavente

In addition to the website mentioned by Dr. Benavente, you can read up on the clinical trials of *LifeOne* and order the product at: *LifeOne.org*.

Protocel: Also known and marketed as *Entelev* and/or *Cancell* it's all the same product, but *Protocel* is the most common name.

Protocel is a unique product that took the inventor, Jim Sheridan, nearly 60 years to perfect. It isn't like the other products, it's not a combination of vitamins, minerals or herbs that each have anticancer properties. *Protocel* is a synergistic combo of all natural and side effect free ingredients that, when taken together as one, destroy cancer cells. Taken individually, only the *Inositol* in it would have anticancer properties all by itself. What's in it, you ask?

- A proprietary blend of Guaiacol, Oil of Vitriol, and Sodium Bromide
- Copper (as Sulfate)
- Inositol
- Potassium
- Sodium

Protocel targets *lower voltage* cells (cancer cells) and acts as a mechanism by which the *voltage* of the cells is lowered even more, to the point where the cancer cells actually break down and turn into harmless proteins. The *voltage* lowering effect of Protocel does not harm healthy cells because those cells have such a high *voltage* in the first place that it does not affect them at all.

There is a very well researched book written by Tanya Harter Pierce called *Outsmart Your Cancer* that gives you all of the details of how Protocel works, and it can be found at *OutsmartYourCancer.com*. If you choose this protocol, this book is **mandatory** reading as it tells you all that you will need to know. The official website of *Protocel* is *Protocel.com*.

Carnivora: This is one of my favorites, for one reason; 19 years before he died (1985) and while he was still in office, Ronald Reagan secretly went to Germany and consulted Germany's leading cancer doctor, Hans Nieper, M.D., concerning his colon cancer and was treated with *Carnivora*, which is a pure extract of the Venus Flytrap plant. I find it amusing that the man sitting in the highest office in America said "screw that" to chemotherapy and radiation. He did have a couple of feet of his colon removed via surgery, but sought alternative treatments thereafter. As a matter of fact, *before* he went to Germany for *Carnivora* treatments he was receiving *laetrile* (active ingredient in **apricot seeds**, remember?) treatments in the oval office for 13 months!

Carnivora is a powerful immune system booster, which stops abnormal growths and kills cancer cells. It is shown to shrink tumors very effectively. *Carnivora* is shown to work for all cancers *except for blood cancers* (leukemia). *Carnivora* has also been used to treat arthritis, lyme disease, hepatitis C, Chrohn's Disease, lupus, chronic fatigue syndrome, ulcerative colitis and multiple sclerosis.

"If I could only choose a single plant medication to use, the answer would be simple: Venus Flytrap. Why Venus Flytrap? In a word, its extract is the most versatile plant-based substance for the treatment of chronic infections and degenerative disease that I have ever experienced."

- Dr. Dan Kenner (*DanKennerResearch.com*)

The venus flytrap plant has over 17 different substances in it that boost immunity:

Droserone: Free radical scavenger.

Hydroplumbagin: Immune Modulation/Stimulation.

Quercetin: Anti-oxidant, free radical scavenger, protectant.

Formic Acid: Natural bactericidal.

Myricetin: Bioflavonoid. Identical properties as Quercetin.

Gallic Acid: Antioxidant, Immune stimulative.

Arginine: Supports NK function. Improves immune responses to foreign entities, crucial for tissue repair.

Asparagine: Explusion of harmful ammonia, increased resistance to fatigue and increase of endurance.

Threonine: Aids in function of intestinal/digestive tracts. Assists in metabolism and assimilation of nutrients; Prevention of fat build-up in the liver.

Glutamine: Helps maintain white blood cell population and T-cell production, supports intestinal health. Nature's brain food to improve mental capacities, decrease fatigue, controls craving for sugar.

Alanine: Strengthens immune system by producing antibodies, important source of energy for muscle tissue, brain and central nervous system.

Cysteine: Facilitates the production of glutathione, which enable white blood cells (lymphocytes such as T cells, B cells and NK cells) to reproduce to make antibodies to destroy foreign substances in the body.

Serine: Component of production of immune antibodies. Antibodies bind with antigens which are toxins, etc. destroying them and removing them from the body.

Histidine: Found abundantly in hemoglobin. This amino acid is used as a potent free-radical scavenger to normalize systemic functions in the body.

Proteases: Known for their ability to enhance immunity, proteases are considered an important line of defense and intestinal toxicity are among the most common symptoms of protease deficiency.

Lipopolysaccharides: Contribute to stimulation of the immune system. Contains properties that are highly potent against harmful cellular entities.

Phytohormones: Plant-derived building blocks that your body can use to rapidly create any hormone that your body needs. These substances, also called phytosterols, are vital to a healthy balanced endocrine or hormonal system.

The developer of *Carnivora*, Dr. Helmut G. Keller, an oncologist from Germany, has more than three decades of lab studies and clinical investigation with over **15,000** cancer patients to back him up.

"In 1973, more than thirty years ago, I discovered why Carnivora is such an effective dietary supplement for the immune system. As you know, this plant is an expert at trapping its own meals through a sensitive biological response process. When a fly or other small insect touches the delicate hairs of the plant's 'mouth,' it causes the mouth to close quickly, trapping the insect inside the plant. The juicy liquids inside the plant's mouth are capable of digesting animal and vegetable materials. Interestingly, they do not, however, digest the plant itself. From this observation, I concluded that the Venus Flytrap plant must have an advanced immune system capable of distinguishing between harmful intruder organisms and its own materials.

In fact, the plant only digests the 'primitive' undeveloped, undifferentiated cells of its own prey. These 'primitive' cells are the same kind of cells that intrude into the human body. These primitive cells will proliferate as a result of chronic stress, exposure to pollutants and poor dietary habits, which the body's immune system is programmed to attack. Supplementing the diet with the seventeen known inherent components of Carnivora supports the immune system multi-dimensionally by fortifying the body's own defense mechanisms."

- Dr. Helmut G. Keller

You can engage in further research and purchase this product at Dr. Keller's website: *Carnivora.com*.

Protandim: Protandim is a synergistic blend of five different herbs (ashwagandha, bacopa, turmeric, green tea and milk thistle) which acts as a "super free radical fighter". Protandim stimulates the production of the free radical fighting enzymes dismutase, catalase and glutathione. By stimulating the production of these enzymes the body's ability to fight off free radicals is massively increased because these enzymes are far more powerful than standard antioxidants.

"Common antioxidants are very limited in their abilities, and in truth they only offer benefits outside the antioxidant realm. The body's enzymes, however, can each eliminate approximately one million free radicals per second without being used up. The advantage of enzymes over antioxidant vitamins is almost mind blowing."

- Dr. Joe McCord

These free radical fighting enzymes have been shown to reduce tumors, slow down cancer cell reproduction and decrease inflammation. *Louisiana State University* researchers, Dr. Jianfeng Lui and assistants, published a study on the cancer fighting properties of *Protandim* in 2009 entitled *"Protandim, a Fundamentally New Antioxidant Approach in Chemoprevention Using Mause Two-Stage Skin Carcinogens as a Model"* and can be read at the following link:
http://journals.plos.org/plosone/article?id=10.1371/journal.pone.0005284

Many other universities and institutions have published studies on *Protandim* as well. I personally wouldn't use *Protandim by itself* as a cancer treatment, but clearly it would be a powerful *addition* to my cancer fighting arsenal. *Protandim* can be purchased and further personal research concerning the scientific studies can be done at *Protandim.com*.

Sea Cucumber: *Sea Cucumber* is a relative of the starfish that lives in all parts of the world deep in the ocean. Being naturally high in chondroitin sulfate and other important nutrients it has been used in Chinese medicine for centuries as a source of joint health. Recently other extraordinary uses of *Sea Cucumber* have been discovered. In a study done at *Robert H. Lurie Cancer Center* in Chicago in 2011, they found that *Sea Cucumber* kills cancer cells within 5 minutes of exposure to the extract. Pancreatic cancer cells were destroyed almost immediately. Additionally, *Sea Cucumber* is effective at combating lung cancer, colon cancer, skin cancer, prostate cancer, liver cancer, breast cancer and others. *Sea Cucumber* also stimulates the immune system and activates its killer cells, which gives it even more cancer combating power. *Sea Cucumber* can be purchased at virtually any health food store.

Selenium: Yes, just good old selenium. Believe it or not, *selenium is perhaps the most potent cancer fighter in nature*. Numerous studies in humans (which can be found at *Scholar.Google.com* by typing in "selenium cancer") have shown selenium to be effective at holding off various types of cancer including breast, stomach, esophageal, prostate, liver and bladder. If you're not taking a selenium supplement, you need to, because the studies show that *the higher the levels of selenium, the lower the levels of cancer.* A worldwide study done by Dr. Gerhard Schrauzer, M.D., Ph.D. from the *University of California* looked at the blood banks of 27 countries, and it showed that the ones with the lowest selenium levels had the highest rates of cancer. And of course, the ones with the highest selenium levels had the lowest rates of cancer.

"If every man, woman and child supplemented with 200 mcg of selenium, we could almost wipe out the cancer epidemic over night!"

- Ty Bollinger, author of *Cancer: Step Outside the Box*

Ellagic acid: Ellagic acid can be found in about 50 different fruits (strawberries, raspberries, blueberries, grapes, pomegranates) and also in walnuts. The *Hollings Cancer Institute* at the *University of South Carolina* conducted a nine year *double blind study* on 500 cervical cancer patients which was published in 1999. It showed that ellagic acid (primarily from raspberries) stops cell division within 48 hours and promotes cellular suicide (apoptosis) of cancer cells within 72 hours for cancers including breast, pancreas, colon, skin, prostate and esophageal. Ellagic acid supplements can be purchased at virtually any health food store.

Inositol: *Inositol* is a naturally occurring substance found in seeds, bran, whole grains, and legumes. It kills cancer cells by stealing iron from them, effectively taking away their primary source of growth. Iron is needed to produce new DNA by cancer cells. Don't worry, inositol doesn't steal iron from healthy cells because, unlike cancer cells, they are tightly bound with hemoglobin. *Inositol* also activates the killer cells of the immune system and reduces tumor sizes. This is just another example of the power of nature to combat cancer, and another fine piece of ammo for your arsenal. *Inositol* supplements can be purchased at virtually any health food store.

Melatonin: Melatonin is a hormone produced naturally in the brain by the pineal gland, mainly at night, when it starts getting dark. *Melatonin* is one of the very best natural sleep aids, and it's why you get sleepy at night. But just as important is the fact that not only is melatonin a free radical fighter and an immune system booster, numerous studies have shown that it also *kills cancer cells*. Dr. David E. Blask, in his report to the *American Association for Cancer Research*, reported that melatonin "puts breast cancer cells to sleep" and also pointed out that it slows breast cancer growth by 70%. *Melatonin* is also reported to shrink many different types of cancerous tumors and is shown to induce cellular suicide (apoptosis) of cancerous cells as well. *Melatonin* supplements can be purchased at any health food store, and a great natural source of melatonin is *cherries*.

DMSO: *DMSO* is a naturally occurring substance found in fruits, vegetables, milk, wheat grass, and aloe vera. In the 1960s a team of scientists at the *University of Oregon* conducted a study where *DMSO* was combined with a purple die and injected into patients with cancer. They did that to find out which cells were affected by the *DMSO*. Their findings were that *DMSO* is attracted to cancerous cells. Not only that, some of the patients were inadvertently *cured* of their cancer during the study!

Source: *"Haematoxylon [a dye] Dissolved in Dimethylsulfoxide [DMSO] Used in Recurrent Neoplasms [i.e. cancer cells or tumor cells]"* by E. J. Tucker, M.D., F.A.C.S., and A. Carrizo, M.D. in *International Surgery*, June 1968, Vol 49, No. 6, page 516.

Cesium Chloride: Cesium chloride therapy is one of the most popular treatments for terminal patients that have been sent home to die from mainstream "doctors". It has been very popular in alternative medicine for over thirty years. This protocol is extremely powerful and when it comes to cancers that have spread significantly, to the bones and other areas of the body, it's one of the most proven cancer therapies, period. Other therapies aren't so powerful when it comes to advanced cancers. **This one is**. Because it is so powerful, it does come with safety warnings, but if you've been sent home to die by mainstream "medicine" and other alternative treatments aren't powerful enough, are the safety warnings really warranted? If you have a choice between death and cesium chloride therapy, are you going to choose death? Probably not.

One very successful practitioner of the cesium chloride therapy was none other than Hans Nieper, M.D., the doctor mentioned above who treated Ronald Reagan with *Carnivora*. Commonly used in conjunction with *DMSO* therapy, cesium chloride is a highly alkaline mineral, which raises the pH of the body in similar fashion to the "baking soda cure". If you remember the quote above from Dr. Otto Warburg, the discoverer of cancer in 1931, he said *"No disease, including cancer, can exist in an alkaline environment"*. Not only does the alkalinity of cesium chloride effectively kill cancer cells, it also limits the intake of glucose into the cancerous cells, depriving it of its favorite food source; sugar. Additionally, it effectively neutralizes lactic acid, which is what causes the uncontrollable multiplication of the cancerous cells. So, as you can see, we have a multiple weapon here against cancer, which is why it is so effective. There are multiple studies that came up for me on *Scholar.Google.com* when I inquired with a "cesium chloride cancer" search. More in depth information concerning this protocol can be seen at the *CancerTutor.com* website: http://www.cancertutor.com/alkaline

Herbs and their Essential Oils: At this point your brain might be on overload, especially if all of this is new to you. After reading about so many different herbs and nutritional substances that fight cancer you might be wondering "How many are there?" I know I was. The answer is that there are probably too many to count. Cancer fighting substances in nature are all over the place, and as if I haven't shown you enough already I'd like to end this section with a massive list of herbs and their essential oils that are proven to have anticancer properties. I did a *Scholar.Google.com* search for the majority of these, and did find studies backing them up for cancer fighting potential. I also found this interesting article from the *American Journal of Cancer Research* entitled *"Anticancer activity of essential oils and their chemical components - a review"*:

"Essential oils are widely used in pharmaceutical, sanitary, cosmetic, agriculture and food industries for their bactericidal, virucidal, fungicidal, antiparasitical and insecticidal properties. Their anticancer activity is well documented. Over a hundred essential oils from more than twenty plant families have been tested on more than twenty types of cancers in last ten years. This review is focused on the activity of essential oils and their components on various types of cancers."

Full article is here: *http://www.ncbi.nlm.nih.gov/pmc/articles/PMC4266698/*

So are you ready for the list? OK. The following herbs and their essential oils do, in fact, demonstrate anticancer potential in laboratory studies. Simply type them in on *Scholar.Google.com* followed by the word "cancer" and see for yourself. Keep in mind what I said earlier, that there are probably too many cancer fighting substances in nature to count. This list of 100 herbs and essential oils is far from complete:

- Allspice
- Aloe aborescens
- Aloe vera
- Angelica
- Anise
- Ammania
- Apple Seeds
- Apricot Seeds
- Artemisia (Wormwood)
- Asafoetida
- Ashwagandha
- Bacopa
- Balsam Fir
- Baptisia
- Barberry
- Black Pepper
- Benzoin
- Bergamot
- Bitter Melon
- Blackberry Bush
- Black Walnut Hulls
- Blackberry
- Blepharis edulis
- Blood Orange
- Boswellia serrata (Frankincense)
- Buckthorn
- Burdock root
- Cacao
- Camphor
- Cannabis
- Cardamom
- Cascara
- Cat's Claw
- Cayenne
- Chamomile
- Chaparral
- Clove
- Coriander
- Dandelion
- Davana
- Dioscorea
- Echinacea
- Eucalyptus

- Foxglove
- Galbanum
- Garlic
- Gentian
- Geranium
- Ginger Root
- Ginseng
- Goldenseal
- Graviola
- Grape Seed
- Green Tea
- Guava
- Helichrysum
- Himalayan Rhubarb
- Hyssop
- Indian Sarsaparilla
- Jasmine
- Lemongrass
- Lepidium sativum (Garden Cress)
- Liquorice Root
- Medicinal Mushrooms
- Milk Thistle
- Mistletoe
- Myrrh
- Nightshades
- Oldenlandia
- Oleander
- Onion
- Oregano
- Passion Flower
- Patchouli
- Poke Root
- Polygala senega
- Red Clover
- Rosemary
- Rue
- Saffron
- Sandalwood
- Scrophularia
- Scutellaria barbata (Skullcap)
- Sheep's Sorrel
- Slippery Elm Bark
- Smilax china
- Stillingia
- Tea Tree Oil
- Thuja
- Thyme
- Tribulus
- Turkey Tail Fungus
- Turkish Rhubarb
- Turmeric (Curcumin)
- Venus Fly Trap
- White Cedar
- White Lily (Lilium album)
- Wintergreen
- Yarrow
- Ysuga

After writing this chapter on cancer, which turned out to be about five times longer than I thought it would be, I can't help but cringe when I think about the fact that when someone gets cancer the "medical profession" tells them that surgery, chemotherapy and radiation are their "only options". The words "hurry, let's poison you to death as quickly as possible" come to mind, as the cancer industry rolls in $200 billion+ in profits every year. That is simply unacceptable, and mere words cannot express how upset I am about all of that. I'd try to express it, but instead of filling the page with cuss words I think I'll just say that I am terrified by the intentional acts of genocide that are taking place, I am *greatly insulted* and I abhor it at the very deepest level of my soul. To all "doctors" who read this, oncologists in particular: Now that you know about these effective treatments, if you keep prescribing *death* (chemotherapy, radiation) to patients when they get cancer you will pay! I'd say that you'll rot in hell, but I don't believe in hell. I do however, believe in *karma*, and you will get yours, that's guaranteed! If you have a conscience, and if you're a decent person, you'll stop prescribing chemotherapy and radiation immediately upon finishing this book. You will stop participating in the genocide of innocent people and you will do **the right thing**.

If you think I covered all of the known cures and effective treatments for cancer, you thought wrong. I'd have to write a whole separate book to do that. There are many other proven effective treatments; *Intravenous Hydrogen Peroxide Therapy, Intravenous Vitamin C Therapy, Hyperthermia Therapy, Ultraviolet Blood Irradiation Therapy* and others! If you have cancer and want to explore your options, I very highly recommend the book *Cancer: Step Outside the Box* by Ty Bollinger. I also place high emphasis on the website *CancerTutor.com* as it is an invaluable resource which details everything I detailed in this book plus about ten times more!

Conclusion

As I've so eloquently proven in this book, the *American Medical Association*, the *American Cancer Society*, the *American Diabetes Association*, the *US Department of Agriculture*, the *US Food and Drug Administration*, the *World Health Organization*, the *US Centers for Disease Control* and all of the rest of them, **especially the drug companies who are calling the shots and running the show**, have been engaged in and continue to be engaged in totally immoral acts of genocide and mass murder upon the population of common people in the name of corporate interests and profits. The drugs and "treatments" that they sell to the public as "promoting health" do no such thing. They kill and maim and cause more harm than good, especially concerning vaccines, HIV and cancer. They destroy the lives of innocent children with drugs like Ritalin, and they destroy the lives of innocent people with their so-called "antidepressants" which might raise serotonin levels, sure, but school shootings, massive violence and suicidal thoughts are common side effects! The "medical professionals" can do better than this! I'm calling bullshit on their whole system!

As citizenry who are aware of what they are doing it is our responsibility to do two things: **1)** refuse all unnecessary treatments and **use nutritional medicines**, effectively **boycotting** the criminals that are the drug companies and **2) educate** your fellow citizens by passing out leaflets, passing along this book, posting info on networking sites such as FaceBook and Twitter, and so on and so forth. As someone who is now aware of the crimes, it now becomes your duty and responsibility to become outspoken about it, because sitting back and being a silent witness to all of it without saying anything about it is exactly the same thing as saying "it's ok with me, let it continue". **Silence is consent**. So for humanity's sake, get busy, and start passing the word along!

"Everything on the earth has a purpose, every disease an herb to cure it, and every person a mission. This is the Indian theory of existence."

- Mourning Dove

Kenneth C. Dyer, Jr.

Appendix A

23 Studies on Low-Carb and Low-Fat Diets

Source: *http://authoritynutrition.com/23-studies-on-low-carb-and-low-fat-diets*
By Kris Gunnars

All of the studies are randomized controlled trials, the gold standard of science. All are published in respected, peer-reviewed journals. Most of the studies were conducted on people with health problems, including overweight/obesity, type II diabetes and metabolic syndrome. The main outcomes measured are usually weight loss, as well as common risk factors like Total Cholesterol, LDL Cholesterol, HDL Cholesterol, Triglycerides and Blood Sugar levels.

1. Foster GD, et al. A randomized trial of a low-carbohydrate diet for obesity. New England Journal of Medicine, 2003.

Details: 63 individuals were randomized to either a low-fat diet group, or a low-carb diet group. The low-fat group was calorie restricted. This study went on for 12 months.

Weight Loss: The low-carb group lost more weight, 7.3% of total body weight, compared to the low-fat group, which lost 4.5%. The difference was statistically significant at 3 and 6 months, but not 12 months.

Conclusion: There was more weight loss in the low-carb group, significant at 3 and 6 months, but not 12. The low-carb group had greater improvements in blood triglycerides and HDL, but other biomarkers were similar between groups.

2. Samaha FF, et al. A low-carbohydrate as compared with a low-fat diet in severe obesity. New England Journal of Medicine, 2003.

Details: 132 individuals with severe obesity (mean BMI of 43) were randomized to either a low-fat or a low-carb diet. Many of the subjects had metabolic syndrome or type II diabetes. The low-fat dieters were calorie restricted. Study duration was 6 months.

Weight Loss: The low-carb group lost an average of 5.8 kg (12.8 lbs) while the low-fat group lost only 1.9 kg (4.2 lbs). The difference was statistically significant.

Conclusion: The low-carb group lost significantly more weight (about 3 times as much). There was also a statistically significant difference in several biomarkers:

Triglycerides went down by 38 mg/dL in the LC group, compared to 7 mg/dL in the LF group. Insulin sensitivity improved on LC, got slightly worse on LF.

Fasting blood glucose levels went down by 26 mg/dL in the LC group, only 5 mg/dL in the LF group.
Insulin levels went down by 27% in the LC group, but increased slightly in the LF group.

Overall, the low-carb diet had significantly more beneficial effects on weight and key biomarkers in this group of severely obese individuals.

3. Sondike SB, et al. Effects of a low-carbohydrate diet on weight loss and cardiovascular risk factor in overweight adolescents. The Journal of Pediatrics, 2003.

Details: 30 overweight adolescents were randomized to two groups, a low-carb diet group and a low-fat diet group. This study went on for 12 weeks. Neither group was instructed to restrict calories.

Weight Loss: The low-carb group lost 9.9 kg (21.8 lbs), while the low-fat group lost 4.1 kg (9 lbs).

Drugging for "Health": Why the Paradigm Must Change

The difference was statistically significant.

Conclusion: The low-carb group lost significantly more (2.3 times as much) weight and had significant decreases in Triglycerides and Non-HDL cholesterol. Total and LDL cholesterol decreased in the low-fat group only.

4. Brehm BJ, et al. A randomized trial comparing a very low carbohydrate diet and a calorie-restricted low fat diet on body weight and cardiovascular risk factors in healthy women. The Journal of Clinical Endocrinology & Metabolism, 2003.

Details: 53 healthy but obese females were randomized to either a low-fat diet, or a low-carb diet. Low-fat group was calorie restricted. The study went on for 6 months.

Weight Loss: The women in the low-carb group lost an average og 8.5 kg (18.7 lbs), while the low-fat group lost an average of 3.9 kg (8.6 lbs). The difference was statistically significant at 6 months.

Conclusion: The low-carb group lost more weight (2.2 times as much) and had significant reductions in blood triglycerides. HDL improved slightly in both groups.

5. Aude YW, et al. The national cholesterol education program diet vs a diet lower in carbohydrates and higher in protein and monounsaturated fat. Archives of Internal Medicine, 2004.

Details: 60 overweight individuals were randomized to a low-carb diet high in monounsaturated fat, or a low-fat diet based on the National Cholesterol Education Program (NCEP).

Both groups were calorie restricted and the study went on for 12 weeks.

Weight Loss: The low-carb group lost an average of 6.2 kg (13.6 lbs), while the low-fat group lost 3.4 kg (7.5 lbs). The difference was statistically significant.

Conclusion: The low-carb group lost 1.8 times as much weight. There were also several changes in biomarkers that are worth noting:

Waist-to-hip ratio, a marker for abdominal fat. Improved slightly in the LC group, not in the LF group.
Total cholesterol improved in both groups.
Triglycerides went down by 42 mg/dL in the LC group, compared to 15.3 mg/dL in the LF group.
LDL particle size increased by 4.8 nm and percentage of small, dense LDL decreased by 6.1% in the LC group, while there was no significant difference in the LF group.
Overall, the low-carb group lost more weight and had much greater improvements in several important risk factors for cardiovascular disease.

6. Yancy WS Jr, et al. A low-carbohydrate, ketogenic diet versus a low-fat diet to treat obesity and hyperlipidemia. Annals of Internal Medicine, 2004.

Details: 120 overweight individuals with elevated blood lipids were randomized to a low-carb or a low-fat diet. The low-fat group was calorie restricted. Study went on for 24 weeks.

Weight Loss: The low-carb group lost 9.4 kg (20.7 lbs) of their total body weight, compared to 4.8 kg (10.6 lbs) in the low-fat group.

Conclusion: The low-carb group lost significantly more weight and had greater improvements in blood triglycerides and HDL cholesterol.

7. JS Volek, et al. Comparison of energy-restricted very low-carbohydrate and low-fat diets on weight loss and body composition in overweight men and women. Nutrition & Metabolism (London), 2004.

Details: A randomized, crossover trial with 28 overweight/obese individuals. Study went on for 30 days (for women) and 50 days (for men) on each diet, that is a very low-carb diet and a low-fat diet. Both diets were calorie restricted.

Weight Loss: The low-carb group lost significantly more weight, especially the men. This was despite the fact that they ended up eating more calories than the low-fat group.

Conclusion: The low-carb group lost more weight. The men on the low-carb diet lost three times as much abdominal fat as the men on the low-fat diet.

8. Meckling KA, et al. Comparison of a low-fat diet to a low-carbohydrate diet on weight loss, body composition, and risk factors for diabetes and cardiovascular disease in free-living, overweight men and women. The Journal of Clinical Endocrinology & Metabolism, 2004.

Details: 40 overweight individuals were randomized to a low-carb and a low-fat diet for 10 weeks. The calories were matched between groups.

Weight Loss: The low-carb group lost 7.0 kg (15.4 lbs) and the low-fat group lost 6.8 kg (14.9 lbs). The difference was not statistically significant.

Conclusion: Both groups lost a similar amount of weight.

A few other notable differences in biomarkers:

Blood pressure decreased in both groups, both systolic and diastolic.
Total and LDL cholesterol decreased in the LF group only.
Triglycerides decreased in both groups.
HDL cholesterol went up in the LC group, but decreased in the LF group.
Blood sugar went down in both groups, but only the LC group had decreases in insulin levels, indicating improved insulin sensitivity.

9. Nickols-Richardson SM, et al. Perceived hunger is lower and weight loss is greater in overweight premenopausal women consuming a low-carbohydrate/high-protein vs high-carbohydrate/low-fat diet. Journal of the American Dietetic Association, 2005.

Details: 28 overweight premenopausal women consumed either a low-carb or a low-fat diet for 6 weeks. The low-fat group was calorie restricted.

Weight Loss: The women in the low-carb group lost 6.4 kg (14.1 lbs) compared to the low-fat group, which lost 4.2 kg (9.3 lbs). The results were statistically significant.

Conclusion: The low-carb diet caused significantly more weight loss and reduced hunger compared to the low-fat diet.

10. Daly ME, et al. Short-term effects of severe dietary carbohydrate-restriction advice in Type 2 diabetes. Diabetic Medicine, 2006.

Details: 102 patients with Type 2 diabetes were randomized to a low-carb or a low-fat diet for 3 months. The low-fat group was instructed to reduce portion sizes.

Weight Loss: The low-carb group lost 3.55 kg (7.8 lbs), while the low-fat group lost only 0.92 kg (2 lbs). The difference was statistically significant.

Conclusion: The low-carb group lost more weight and had greater improvements in the Total cholesterol/HDL ratio. There was no difference in triglycerides, blood pressure or HbA1c (a marker for blood sugar levels) between groups.

Drugging for "Health": Why the Paradigm Must Change

11. McClernon FJ, et al. The effects of a low-carbohydrate ketogenic diet and a low-fat diet on mood, hunger, and other self-reported symptoms. Obesity (Silver Spring), 2007.

Details: 119 overweight individuals were randomized to a low-carb, ketogenic diet or a calorie restricted low-fat diet for 6 months.

Weight Loss: The low-carb group lost 12.9 kg (28.4 lbs), while the low-fat group lost only 6.7 kg (14.7 lbs).

Conclusion: The low-carb group lost almost twice the weight and experienced less hunger.

12. Gardner CD, et al. Comparison of the Atkins, Zone, Ornish, and LEARN diets for change in weight and related risk factors among overweight premenopausal women: the A TO Z Weight Loss Study. The Journal of The American Medical Association, 2007.

Details: 311 overweight/obese premenopausal women were randomized to 4 diets: A low-carb Atkins diet, a low-fat vegetarian Ornish diet, the Zone diet and the LEARN diet. Zone and LEARN were calorie restricted.

Weight Loss: The Atkins group lost the most weight at 12 months (4.7 kg – 10.3 lbs) compared to Ornish (2.2 kg – 4.9 lbs), Zone (1.6 kg – 3.5 lbs) and LEARN (2.6 kg – 5.7 lbs). However, the difference was not statistically significant at 12 months.

Conclusion: The Atkins group lost the most weight, although the difference was not statistically significant. The Atkins group had the greatest improvements in blood pressure, triglycerides and HDL. LEARN and Ornish (low-fat) had decreases in LDL at 2 months, but then the effects diminished.

13. Halyburton AK, et al. Low- and high-carbohydrate weight-loss diets have similar effects on mood but not cognitive performance. American Journal of Clinical Nutrition, 2007.

Details: 93 overweight/obese individuals were randomized to either a low-carb, high-fat diet or a low-fat, high-carb diet for 8 weeks. Both groups were calorie restricted.

Weight Loss: The low-carb group lost 7.8 kg (17.2 lbs), while the low-fat group lost 6.4 kg (14.1 lbs). The difference was statistically significant.

Conclusion: The low-carb group lost more weight. Both groups had similar improvements in mood, but speed of processing (a measure of cognitive performance) improved further on the low-fat diet.

14. Dyson PA, et al. A low-carbohydrate diet is more effective in reducing body weight than healthy eating in both diabetic and non-diabetic subjects. Diabetic Medicine, 2007.

Details: 13 diabetic and 13 non-diabetic individuals were randomized to a low-carb diet or a "healthy eating" diet that followed the Diabetes UK recommendations (a calorie restricted, low-fat diet). Study went on for 3 months.

Weight Loss: The low-carb group lost 6.9 kg (15.2 lbs), compared to 2.1 kg (4.6 lbs) in the low-fat group.

Conclusion: The low-carb group lost more weight (about 3 times as much). There was no difference in any other marker between groups.

15. Westman EC, et al. The effect of a low-carbohydrate, ketogenic diet versus a low-glycemic index diet on glycemic control in type 2 diabetes mellitus. Nutrion & Metabolism (London), 2008.

Details: 84 individuals with obesity and type 2 diabetes were randomized to a low-carb, ketogenic diet or a calorie restricted low-glycemic diet. The study went on for 24 weeks.

Weight Loss: The low-carb group lost more weight (11.1 kg – 24.4 lbs) compared to the low-glycemic group (6.9 kg – 15.2 lbs).

Conclusion: The low-carb group lost significantly more weight than the low-glycemic group. There were several other important differences:

Hemoglobin A1c went down by 1.5% in the LC group, compared to 0.5% in the low-glycemic group.
HDL cholesterol increased in the LC group only, by 5.6 mg/dL.
Diabetes medications were either reduced or eliminated in 95.2% of the LC group, compared to 62% in the low-glycemic group.
Many other health markers like blood pressure and triglycerides improved in both groups, but the difference between groups was not statistically significant.

16. Shai I, et al. Weight loss with a low-carbohydrate, Mediterranean, or low-fat diet. New England Journal of Medicine, 2008.

Details: 322 obese individuals were randomized to three diets: a low-carb diet, a calorie restricted low-fat diet and a calorie restricted Mediterranean diet. Study went on for 2 years.

Weight Loss: The low-carb group lost 4.7 kg (10.4 lbs), the low-fat group lost 2.9 kg (6.4 lbs) and the Mediterranean diet group lost 4.4 kg (9.7 lbs).

Conclusion: The low-carb group lost more weight than the low-fat group and had greater improvements in HDL cholesterol and triglycerides.

17. Keogh JB, et al. Effects of weight loss from a very-low-carbohydrate diet on endothelial function and markers of cardiovascular disease risk in subjects with abdominal obesity. American Journal of Clinical Nutrition, 2008.

Details: 107 individuals with abdominal obesity were randomized to a low-carb or a low-fat diet. Both groups were calorie restricted and the study went on for 8 weeks.

Weight Loss: The low-carb group lost 7.9% of body weight, compared to the low-fat group which lost 6.5% of body weight.

Conclusion: The low-carb group lost more weight and there was no difference between groups on Flow Mediated Dilation or any other markers of the function of the endothelium (the lining of blood vessels). There was also no difference in common risk factors between groups.

18. Tay J, et al. Metabolic effects of weight loss on a very-low-carbohydrate diet compared with an isocaloric high-carbohydrate diet in abdominally obese subjects. Journal of The American College of Cardiology, 2008.

Details: 88 individuals with abdominal obesity were randomized to a very low-carb or a low-fat diet for 24 weeks. Both diets were calorie restricted.

Weight Loss: The low-carb group lost an average of 11.9 kg (26.2 lbs), while the low-fat group lost 10.1 kg (22.3 lbs). However, the difference was not statistically significant.

Conclusion: The low-carb group lost more weight. Triglycerides, HDL, C-Reactive Protein, Insulin, Insulin Sensitivity and Blood Pressure improved in both groups. Total and LDL cholesterol improved in the low-fat group only.

19. Volek JS, et al. Carbohydrate restriction has a more favorable impact on the metabolic syndrome than a low fat diet. Lipids, 2009.

Drugging for "Health": Why the Paradigm Must Change

Details: 40 subjects with elevated risk factors for cardiovascular disease were randomized to a low-carb or a low-fat diet for 12 weeks. Both groups were calorie restricted.

Weight Loss: The low-carb group lost 10.1 kg (22.3), while the low-fat group lost 5.2 kg (11.5 lbs).

Conclusion: The low-carb group lost almost twice the amount of weight as the low-fat group, despite eating the same amount of calories.

This study is particularly interesting because it matched calories between groups and measured so-called "advanced" lipid markers. Several things are worth noting:

Triglycerides went down by 107 mg/dL on LC, but 36 mg/dL on the LF diet.
HDL cholesterol increased by 4 mg/dL on LC, but went down by 1 mg/dL on LF.
Apolipoprotein B went down by 11 points on LC, but only 2 points on LF.
LDL size increased on LC, but stayed the same on LF.
On the LC diet, the LDL particles partly shifted from small to large (good), while they partly shifted from large to small on LF (bad).

20. Brinkworth GD, et al. Long-term effects of a very-low-carbohydrate weight loss diet compared with an isocaloric low-fat diet after 12 months. American Journal of Clinical Nutrition, 2009.

Details: 118 individuals with abdominal obesity were randomized to a low-carb or a low-fat diet for 1 year. Both diets were calorie restricted.

Weight Loss: The low-carb group lost 14.5 kg (32 lbs), while the low-fat group lost 11.5 kg (25.3 lbs) but the difference was not statistically significant.

Conclusion: The low-carb group had greater decreases in triglycerides and greater increases in both HDL and LDL cholesterol, compared to the low-fat group.

21. Hernandez, et al. Lack of suppression of circulating free fatty acids and hypercholesterolemia during weight loss on a high-fat, low-carbohydrate diet. American Journal of Clinical Nutrition, 2010.

Details: 32 obese adults were randomized to a low-carb or a calorie restricted, low-fat diet for 6 weeks.

Weight Loss: The low-carb group lost 6.2 kg (13.7 lbs) while the low-fat group lost 6.0 kg (13.2 lbs). The difference was not statistically significant.

Conclusion: The low-carb group had greater decreases in triglycerides (43.6 mg/dL) than the low-fat group (26.9 mg/dL). Both LDL and HDL decreased in the low-fat group only.

22. Krebs NF, et al. Efficacy and safety of a high protein, low carbohydrate diet for weight loss in severely obese adolescents. Journal of Pediatrics, 2010.

Details: 46 individuals were randomized to a low-carb or a low-fat diet for 36 weeks. Low-fat group was calorie restricted.

Weight Loss: The low-carb group lost more weight and had greater decreases in BMI than the low-fat group.

Conclusion: The low-carb group had greater reductions in BMI. Various biomarkers improved in both groups, but there was no significant difference between groups.

23. Guldbrand, et al. In type 2 diabetes, randomization to advice to follow a low-carbohydrate

diet transiently improves glycaemic control compared with advice to follow a low-fat diet producing a similar weight loss. Diabetologia, 2012.

Details: 61 individuals with type 2 diabetes were randomized to a low-carb or a low-fat diet for 2 years. Both diets were calorie restricted.

Weight Loss: The low-carb group lost 3.1 kg (6.8 lbs), while the low-fat group lost 3.6 kg (7.9 lbs). The difference was not statistically significant.

Conclusion: There was no difference in weight loss or common risk factors between groups. There was significant improvement in glycemic control at 6 months for the low-carb group, but compliance was poor and the effects diminished at 24 months as individuals had increased their carb intake.

****

The majority of studies achieved statistically significant differences in weight loss (always in favor of low-carb). There are several other factors that are worth noting:

The low-carb groups often lost 2-3 times as much weight as the low-fat groups. In a few instances there was no significant difference.

In most cases, calories were restricted in the low-fat groups, while the low-carb groups could eat as much as they wanted.

When both groups restricted calories, the low-carb dieters still lost more weight, although it was not always significant.

There was only one study where the low-fat group lost more weight although the difference was small (0.5 kg – 1.1 lb) and not statistically significant.

In several of the studies, weight loss was greatest in the beginning. Then people start regaining the weight over time as they abandon the diet.

When the researchers looked at abdominal fat (the unhealthy visceral fat) directly, low-carb diets had a clear advantage.

LDL Cholesterol
Despite the concerns expressed by many people, low-carb diets generally do not raise Total and LDL cholesterol levels on average.

Low-fat diets do lower Total and LDL cholesterol, but it is usually only temporary. After 6 to 12 months, the difference is not statistically significant.

There have been some anecdotal reports by doctors who treat patients with low-carb diets, that they can lead to increases in LDL cholesterol and some advanced lipid markers for a small percentage of individuals.

However, none of the studies above noted such adverse effects. The few studies that looked at advanced lipid markers only showed improvements.

HDL Cholesterol
One of the best ways to raise HDL cholesterol levels is to eat more fat. For this reason, it is not surprising to see that low-carb diets (higher in fat) raise HDL significantly more than low-fat diets.

Having higher HDL levels is correlated with improved metabolic health and a lower risk of cardiovascular disease. Having low HDL levels is one of the key symptoms of the metabolic syndrome.

Drugging for "Health": Why the Paradigm Must Change

18 of the 23 studies reported changes in HDL cholesterol levels:

You can see that low-carb diets generally raise HDL levels, while they don't change as much on low-fat diets and in some cases go down.
Triglycerides

Triglycerides are an important cardiovascular risk factor and another key symptom of the metabolic syndrome.

The best way to reduce triglycerides is to eat less carbohydrates, especially sugar.

19 of 23 studies reported changes in blood triglyceride levels:

It is clear that both low-carb and low-fat diets lead to reductions in triglycerides, but the effect is much stronger in the low-carb groups.

Blood Sugar, Insulin Levels and Type II Diabetes
In non-diabetics, blood sugar and insulin levels improved on both low-carb and low-fat diets and the difference between groups was usually small.

3 studies compared low-carb and low-fat diets in Type 2 diabetic patients.

Only one of those studies had good compliance and managed to reduce carbohydrates sufficiently. This lead various improvements and a drastic reduction in HbA1c, a marker for blood sugar levels.

In this study, over 90% of the individuals in the low-carb group managed to reduce or eliminate their diabetes medications.

However, the difference was small or nonexistent in the other two studies, because compliance was poor and the individuals ended up eating carbs at about 30% of calories.

Blood Pressure
When measured, blood pressure tended to decrease on both low-carb and low-fat diets.

Adverse Effects?
Despite the concerns expressed by many health experts in the past, there were zero reports of serious adverse effects that were attributable to either diet.

Overall, the low-carb diet was well tolerated and had an outstanding safety profile.

Keep in mind that all of these studies are randomized controlled trials, the gold standard of science. All are published in respected, peer-reviewed medical journals.

These studies are scientific evidence, as good as it gets, that low-carb is much more effective than the low-fat diet that is still being recommended all over the world.

Appendix B

What Is Reiki? What If I'm Skeptical?

Reiki originated in Japan with Dr. Mikao Usui. It is one of many different modalities of "energy healing." Reiki is not connected with the medical field, it is holistic healing and a Reiki practitioner is not a doctor or a medical professional, nor is Reiki intended to be a replacement for medical treatment. The word Reiki comes from the Japanese word "Rei" which means "Universal Life" and "Ki" which means "Energy." Being quite similar but much more gentle than acupressure or acupuncture, Reiki Masters work with the chakras and meridians of the electromagnetic energy field (aura) of the physical body. It is administered by "laying on hands" but touch is not necessary, it can be done either directly on the body, just above the body or via long distances. Energy healing is based upon Einstein's scientifically proven fact that we are all made of nothing but pure electromagnetic energy. All matter is composed of atoms, and all atoms are composed of electrically charged particles (protons, neutrons and electrons) which interact magnetically with each other. The protons and neutrons make up the nucleus of the atom in the center, while the electrons travel around the nucleus similar to the way that the earth travels around the sun. The electromagnetism of the nucleus is what keeps the electrons traveling in circles. Our bodies function the same way, on a larger scale. We are all bodies of light and electromagnetic energy. Nothing is solid. Everyone has an aura. We also have seven main chakra points that correspond in color to the colors on the electromagnetic spectrum, basically the seven colors of the rainbow. Our aura, which is an egg shaped body of light that surrounds us, tends to have one dominate color but depending on what's going on in our lives it can also be composed of several different colors. It has also been scientifically proven that the dominate color in our aura changes when our emotions change, and as we go thru our day. Positive thoughts and positive energy literally heal physical illnesses. If your aura contains too many negative vibrations, or if you think too many negative thoughts, then you are more likely to get physically and mentally ill or feel stress, and if you are high in positive energy and positive thoughts, you are more capable of being happy and healthy. What I do as a healer is remove negative energies and replace them with positive energies. I also remove blockages in the flow of energy through the chakra system.

Reiki promotes relaxation, emotional and physical healing, spiritual and personal growth and recovery and addresses all levels of mind, body and spirit. As a person who was once very alienated from people, depressed and generally stressed on life, I can attest that it has completely changed my life and has been nothing short of a miracle for me. I feel that Reiki has saved my life. It also works in conjunction with and is a very nice compliment to all other medical or therapeutic techniques to relieve side effects and promote recovery.

When applying Reiki people often tell me that my hands feel like a heating pad, and they report tingling sensations and a very comfortable state of relaxation. Many have reported miraculous results:

One example of my personal successes was when a co-worker had a shoulder that hurt so badly that he couldn't raise his arm above his head. His condition was like that for one full year and had been seen by medical doctors. During a slow period at work one night, I casually did Reiki on him for about fifteen minutes. The next day he came into work waving his arm around above his head and told me there was only very minimal pain. Fifteen minutes of Reiki cured a one year old shoulder problem that medical doctors were unable to fix.

Another example is a life-long friend of mine, Steve, who had suffered from severe back pain. He had been to doctors for years and had been taking heavy narcotic pain medications daily. Nothing was helping. I talked him into coming to my free Reiki circle, he came limping in like an old man and it took him much effort just to get onto the massage table. He was a hurting unit. I did a full one hour treatment on him for three consecutive Sundays, and by the fourth week he was giving me credit for literally "curing" his back pain. He is now a very serious Reiki Master and goes out playing basketball, does yard work, etc. and says that Reiki has been a miracle in his life and changed his whole perspective.

Reiki Masters intuitively tune into the energy of the aura and use various methods of psychic ability and intuition to guide their healings. Different Reiki Masters have different psychic gifts. Some, like myself, are empathic and feel people's energy. We feel the client's headache like it's our own headache. Or back ache, neck ache, emotional pain, stress, happiness, etc. whatever the person might be feeling. Some of us, including myself, are clairaudient and can hear things like people's thoughts, messages from our spirit guides, the client's spirit guides, the Reiki guides, the client's deceased relatives, and so on and so forth. Some of us are clairvoyant and some just have an inner knowing about things. Everyone has psychic gifts, it is just a matter of unlocking them by ridding yourself of negative energy (baggage) from the past because negative energy and stored pain from the past block intuitive abilities. That is why many of us had experiences as children with psychic abilities but no longer have them. As we grew older the baggage began to accumulate and the abilities started to dissipate. The more you purify your aura, the more you let go of pain from the past, the more intuitive you'll become once again. We can all develop these abilities if we work on healing ourselves of past pain, and Reiki is a very effective way to accomplish that.

Drugging for "Health": Why the Paradigm Must Change

While Reiki is spiritual in nature, it is not a religion. People from all different walks of life and religions practice Reiki. It has no dogma. There is nothing you must believe in order to learn and use Reiki, however if you are a skeptic and are closed off to the possibility of it producing results, then that can and will hinder or perhaps even prevent it from working at all. Just be open minded and all is good.

Dr. Mikao Usui, the founder modern Reiki, created a list of ethics, not "commandments" or dogma but a general set of guidelines which apply to pretty much everyone who wishes to live a clean and peaceful life:

"Just for Today:

I will not worry.

I will not anger.

I will do my work honestly.

I will be kind to every living thing.

I will give thanks for my many blessings.

What If I'm SKEPTICAL?

One of the first things that I recommend for skeptics is that they experience it for themselves. Reiki is a scientifically proven concept, and the only thing can cause it to *not* work is if the recipient is simply so closed minded and skeptical that they will not allow the energy to penetrate their aura. Closed mindedness breeds ineffectiveness when it comes to energy healing, but that's not because energy healing isn't effective. As long as the recipient is at least open minded enough to be open to the *possibility* of it being effective, then it will be effective!

If you require research and scientific evidence of the benefits of Reiki (and other modalities of energy healing) I very highly recommend the following book: *"The Energy Healing Experiments: Science Reveals Our Natural Power to Heal"* which details numerous laboratory experiments, all of which conclusively prove the effectiveness of energy healing. After looking at these individual experiments as well as all of them combined, there is simply no doubting the effectiveness of energy healing. It is definitely a fully fledged scientifically proven concept. The author is Dr. Gary Schwartz, PhD, a professor of psychology, surgery, medicine, neurology and psychiatry at the University of Arizona. He received his PhD from Harvard University and was a professor of psychiatry and psychology at Yale University as well as Director of the Yale Psychophysiology Center and co-director of the Yale Behavioral Medicine Clinic from 1976-1988. He is currently the Director of the Laboratory for Advances in Consciousness and Health in the Department of Psychology at the University of Arizona.

Appendix C

I recommend that you use either Stevia, Monk Fruit Extract or Erythritol for sweeteners. They are all natural and side effect free and can be found at most health food stores. I personally like to drink an all natural soda every now and then; there is an all natural sugar free brand available in most health food stores called "Zevia" that uses all three sweeteners mentioned above and the natural ingredients give it far more flavor than the mainstream diet sodas, it tastes really good.

Other low calorie sweeteners like Splenda, Saccharin and Sweet 'n Low are just as bad as Aspartame, they aren't natural and studies show that all three cause cancer in mice.

Aspartame Side Effects
Source: *http://www.sweetpoison.com/aspartame-side-effects.html*

Written by Janet Starr Hull, author of *"Sweet Poison"*

There are over 92 different health side effects associated with aspartame consumption. It seems surreal, but true. How can one chemical create such chaos?

Aspartame dissolves into solution and can therefore travel throughout the body and deposit within any tissue. The body digests aspartame unlike saccharin, which does not break down within humans.

The multitude of aspartame side effects are indicative to your genetic individuality and physical weaknesses. It is important to put two and two together, nonetheless, and identify which side effects aspartame is creating within you.

The components of aspartame can lead to a number of health problems, as you have read. Side effects can occur gradually, can be immediate, or can be acute reactions.

According to Lendon Smith, M.D. there is an enormous population suffering from side effects associated with aspartame, yet have no idea why drugs, supplements and herbs don't relieve their symptoms. Then, there are users who don't 'appear' to suffer immediate reactions at all. Even these individuals are susceptible to the long-term damage caused by excitatory amino acids, phenylalanine, methanol, and DKP.

Adverse reactions and side effects of aspartame include:

Eye
blindness in one or both eyes
decreased vision and/or other eye problems such as: blurring, bright flashes, squiggly lines, tunnel vision, decreased night vision
pain in one or both eyes
decreased tears
trouble with contact lenses
bulging eyes

Ear
tinnitus - ringing or buzzing sound
severe intolerance of noise
marked hearing impairment

Neurologic
epileptic seizures
headaches, migraines and (some severe)
dizziness, unsteadiness, both
confusion, memory loss, both
severe drowsiness and sleepiness

paresthesia or numbness of the limbs
severe slurring of speech
severe hyperactivity and restless legs
atypical facial pain
severe tremors

Psychological/Psychiatric

severe depression
irritability
aggression
anxiety
personality changes
insomnia
phobias

Chest

palpitations, tachycardia
shortness of breath
recent high blood pressure

Gastrointestinal

nausea
diarrhea, sometimes with blood in stools
abdominal pain
pain when swallowing

Skin and Allergies

itching without a rash
lip and mouth reactions
hives
aggravated respiratory allergies such as asthma

Endocrine and Metabolic

loss of control of diabetes
menstrual changes
marked thinning or loss of hair
marked weight loss
gradual weight gain
aggravated low blood sugar (hypoglycemia)
severe PMS

Other

frequency of voiding and burning during urination
excessive thirst, fluid retention, leg swelling, and bloating
increased susceptibility to infection

Additional Symptoms of Aspartame Toxicity include the most critical symptoms of all

death
irreversible brain damage
birth defects, including mental retardation
peptic ulcers
aspartame addiction and increased craving for sweets
hyperactivity in children
severe depression
aggressive behavior
suicidal tendencies

Aspartame may trigger, mimic, or cause the following illnesses:
Chronic Fatigue Syndrome
Epstein-Barr
Post-Polio Syndrome
Lyme Disease
Grave's Disease
Meniere's Disease
Alzheimer's Disease
ALS
Epilepsy
Multiple Sclerosis (MS)
EMS
Hypothyroidism
Mercury sensitivity from Amalgam fillings
Fibromyalgia
Lupus
non-Hodgkins
Lymphoma
Attention Deficit Disorder (ADD)

These are not allergies or sensitivities, but diseases and disease syndromes. Aspartame poisoning is commonly misdiagnosed because aspartame symptoms mock textbook 'disease' symptoms, such as Grave's Disease.

Aspartame changes the ratio of amino acids in the blood, blocking or lowering the levels of serotonin, tyrosine, dopamine, norepinephrine, and adrenaline. Therefore, it is typical that aspartame symptoms cannot be detected in lab tests and on x-rays. Textbook disorders and diseases may actually be a toxic load as a result of aspartame poisoning.

Ever gone to the doctor with real, physical symptoms, but he/she can't find the cause? Well, it's probably your diet, your environment, or both.

Aspartame is the common denominator for over 92 different health symptoms at the root of modern disease. The Aspartame Detoxification Program demonstrates the most effective way to reverse disease symptoms is removing the underlying cause - aspartame.

I counsel aspartame victims worldwide and have witnessed nine out of 10 clients restore their health by following the Aspartame Detoxification Program. Begin with detoxifying your body of all residual chemical toxins from aspartame's chemical make up of phenylalanine, aspartic acid and methanol and their toxic by-products, and see if any adverse health symptoms remain. Try the Aspartame Detoxification Program, and within 30 days your symptoms should disappear.

Steps:

Remove all sugar-free products with aspartame from your diet.
Learn to 'read' your body. Begin recording any health changes.
Get a hair analysis.
Be happy with yourself.
Detoxify.
Restore depleted nutrients.
Exercise and get plenty of rest.
Eat 75% raw foods at every meal.
Drink water, water, water.
Get control of your life.
I designed this Ten Step Program to help protect your health and the health of those you love from being seduced by the sugar-free diet craze. Wishing you good health.

Suggested Reading

ADD/ADHD

ADHD Does Not Exist: The Truth About Attention Deficit and Hyperactivity Disorder by Richard Saul

No More Ritalin by Dr. Mary Ann Block

Not My Kid: A Parent's Guide to Kids and Drugs by Beth Polson & Miller Newton

The A.D.D. Nutrition Solution: A Drug-Free 30 Day Plan by Marcia Zimmerman

The ADD and ADHD Cure: The Natural Way to Treat Hyperactivity and Refocus Your Child by Jay Gordon, M.D. with Jennifer Chang

Alzheimers/Dementia

Mind Boosters: Natural Supplements That Enhance Mind, Memory, and Mood by Ray Sahelian, M.D.

Arthritis

Healing Joint Pain Naturally by Ellen Hodgson Brown

The Inflammation Syndrome: Your Nutrition Plan for Great Health, Weight Loss, and Pain-Free Living by Jack Challem

Aspartame/Artifical Sweeteners

Sweet Poison by Janet Starr Hull

Cancer

A Cancer Therapy: Results of Fifty Cases and the Cure of Advanced Cancer by Dr. Max Gerson

Alive and Well: One Doctor's Experience With Nutrition in the Treatment of Cancer Patients by Philip E. Binzel, Jr., M.D.

Beating Cancer Gently by Dr. Bill Henderson

Cancer: Curing the Incurable Without Surgery, Chemotherapy or Radiation by Dr. William Donald Kelley

Cancer is a Fungus by Dr. Tullio Simoncini

Cancer: Its Cause and Its Cure by Dr. Otto Warburg

Cancer: Step Outside the Box by Ty Bollinger

Doctored Results: The Suppression of Laetrile at Sloan-Kettering Institute for Cancer Research by Ralph W. Moss

Knockout: Interviews With Doctors Who Are Curing Cancer and How To Prevent Getting It In the First Place by Suzanne Summers

Marijuana Killed My Cancer and is keeping me cancer free: Step-by-step guide how to kill your cancer with cannabis The healing miracle of CBD plus THC by Erika M. Karohs Ph.D.

Natures Answer For Cancer by Rick Simpson

Outsmart Your Cancer by Tanya Harter Pierce

The Cancer Cure That Worked by Barry Lynes

The Definitive Guide to Cancer: An Integrative Approach to Prevention, Treatment, and Healing by Lise N. Alschuler & Karolyn A. Gazella

The Enzyme Theory of Cancer by Dr. John Beard

The Healing of Cancer by Barry Lynes

The Politics of Cancer by Dr. Samuel Epstein

When Healing Becomes a Crime: The Amazing Story of the Hoxsey Cancer Clinics by Kenny Ausubel

Cannabis

Cannabis Pharmacy: The Practical Guide to Medical Marijuana by Michael Backes

Marihuana Reconsidered by Lester Grinspoon, M.D.

Smoke Signals: A Social History of Marijuana - Medical, Recreational and Scientific by Martin A. Lee

Cholesterol

The Great Cholesterol Con by Dr. Malcolm Kendrick, M.D.

The Great Cholesterol Myth: Why Lowering Your Cholesterol Won't Prevent Heart Disease-and the Statin-Free Plan That Will by Jonny Bowden, Ph.D., C.N.S.

Depression

5-HTP: The Natural Way to Overcome Depression, Obesity, and Insomnia by Dr. Michael Murray, N.D.

Stop Depression Now: SAM-e: The Breakthrough Supplement that Works as Well as Prescription Drugs by Richard Brown & Carol Colman

The Depression Cure: The 11-Step Program to Naturally Beat Depression For Life by Tai Morello

The Natural Medicine Guide to Bipolar Disorder by Stephanie Marohn

Diabetes

Atkins Diabetes Revolution: The Groundbreaking Approach To Preventing and Controlling Type 2 Diabetes by Mary C. Vernon M.D., C.M.D. & Jacqueline A. Eberstein, R.N.

Drugging for "Health": Why the Paradigm Must Change

Reversing Diabetes by Julian Whitaker

The New Glucose Revolution: Low GI Eating Made Easy by Dr. Jennie Brand-Miller M.D. M.D. & Kaye Foster-Powell M. Nutr & Diet

The Sugar Solution: Balance Your Blood Sugar Naturally to Avoid Disease, Lose Weight, Gain Energy, and Feel Great by Sarí Harrar (Editor) & Julia Vantine (Editor)

Electromedicine

Cross Currents: The Promise of Electromedicine, The Perils of Electropollution by Dr. Robert O. Becker

The Body Electric: Electromagnetism and the Foundation of Life by Dr. Robert O. Becker

Energy Medicine

Essential Reiki by Dianne Stein

Hands of Light by Barbara Brennen

Matrix Energetics: The Science and Art of Transformation by Richard Bartlett, D.C., N.D.

The Energy Healing Experiments: Science Reveals Our Natural Power to Heal by Gary E. Schwartz Ph.D.

General Awareness/New World Order

Human Race Get Off Your Knees: The Lion Sleeps No More by David Icke

Monumental Myths of the Modern Medical Mafia by Ty Bollinger

Official Stories by Liam Scheff

The Perception Deception by David Icke

General Expose' of the Medical System

Bad Pharma: How Drug Companies Mislead Doctors and Harm Patients by Ben Goldacre

General Health/Herbs/Supplements/Nutrition

Barefoot on Coral Calcium: "An Elixir of Life" Health Secrets of the Coral of Okinawa by Robert R. Barefoot

Dr. Atkins Vita-Nutrient Solution: Nature's Answer to Drugs by Dr. Robert C. Atkins, M.D.

Dr. Atkins' Age Defying Diet Revolution by Robert C. Atkins, M.D.

Herbal Antibiotics by Steven Harrod Buhner

Herbal Antivirals by Steven Harrod Buhner

Herbal Prescriptions for Better Health by Dr. Donald J. Brown, N.D.

Naturopathic Handbook of Herbal Formulas: A Practical and Concise Herb User's Guide by Herbal Research Publications, Inc.

Natural Health, Natural Medicine by Andrew Weil, M.D.

Prescription for Natural Cures by Dr. James F. Balch, M.D.

Prescription for Nutritional Healing by Phyllis A. Balch, C.N.C.

Radical Healing by Rudolph Ballentine, M.D.

The Coconut Oil Miracle by Bruce Fife, C.N., M.D.

The Encyclopedia of Natural Medicine by Michael T. Murray, N.D.

The Herbal Drugstore by Linda B. White, M.D.

The New Healing Herbs by Michael Castleman

The Omega RX Zone: The Miracle of the New High Dose Fish Oil by Dr. Barry Sears

The Pill Book Guide to Natural Medicine by Dr. Michael Murray, N.D.

The Whole Truth About Spirulina: Documented Results by Users and Health Care Professionals No Author Indicated

Total Wellness by Joseph Pizzorno, N.D.

Water: For Health, for Healing, for Life: You're Not Sick, You're Thirsty! by F. Batmanghelidj

What The Drug Companies Won't Tell You and Your Doctor Doesn't Know by Michael T. Murray, N.D.

What Your Doctor Doesn't Know About Nutritional Medicine May Be Killing You by Ray D. Strand

HIV/AIDS

AIDS: The HIV Myth by Jad Adams

Deadly Deception: The Proof That SEX and HIV Absolutely DO NOT Cause AIDS by Robert E. Wilner, M.D., Ph.D.

Infectious AIDS: Have We Been Mislead? by Peter H. Duesberg

Inventing the AIDS Virus by Peter H. Duesberg

The Great AIDS Hoax by T.C. Fry

What If Everything You Thought You Knew About AIDS Was Wrong? by Christine Maggiore

Low Carb Diet

Dr. Atkins New Diet Revolution by Dr. Robert C. Atkins, M.D.

Good Calories, Bad Calories by Gary Taubes

Life Without Bread: How a Low Carb Diet Can Save Your Life by Christian B. Allen, Ph.D. & Wolfgang Lutz, M.D.

Drugging for "Health": Why the Paradigm Must Change

Living Low Carb by Jonny Bowden, Ph.D., C.N.S.

Wheat Belly by William Davis, M.D.

Prescription Drug Hazards

Overdosed America: The Broken Promise of American Medicine by John Abramson

The Risks of Prescription Drugs by Donald W. Light

Thyroid/Adrenal/Endrocrine System Health

Adrenal Fatigue Syndrome: Reclaim your Energy and Vitality with Clinically Proven Natural Programs by Michael Lam & Dorine Lam

Living Well With Hypothyroidism by Mary J. Shomon

Stop the Thyroid Madness by Janie A. Bowthorpe, M.Ed.

Stop the Thyroid Madness II by Janie A. Bowthorpe, M.Ed

The Cortisol Connection by Shawn Talbott, Ph.D.

The Thyroid Diet by Mary J. Shomon

Thyroid Power: 10 Steps to Total Health by Richard L. Shames, M.D. & Karilee Halo Shames, R.N., Ph.D.

Vaccines

Bypassing Bypass: The New Technique of Chelation Therapy by Elmer Cranton, Arline Brecher & James P. Frackelton

Immunization: The Reality Behind the Myth by Walene James

The Chelation Way: The Complete Book of Chelation Therapy by Dr. Morton Walker

Vaccine Epidemic: How Corporate Greed, Biased Science, and Coercive Government Threaten Our Human Rights, Our Health, and Our Children by Louise Kuo Habakas, M.A. & Mary Holland, J.D.

Suggested Films/Documentaries

Most of these can be found on *YouTube.com* and viewed for free.

Aspartame

"Sweet Misery: A Poisoned World"

Cancer

"Burzynski the Movie: Cancer Is Serious Business" (parts 1 and 2)

"Cancer: The Forbidden Cures"

"Run From the Cure" (the Rick Simpson Story)

"Second Opinion: Laetrile At Sloan-Kettering"

"World Without Cancer" by G. Edward Griffin

General Expose' of the Medical System

"Bought: The Truth Behind Big Pharma, Vaccines and Your Food" - *BoughtMovie.com*

HIV/AIDS

"HIV=AIDS: FACT or FRAUD"

"House of Numbers"

"The Other Side of AIDS"

New World Order

"The Money Masters"

Vaccines

"Silent Epidemic; The Untold Story of Vaccines"

ABOUT THE AUTHOR

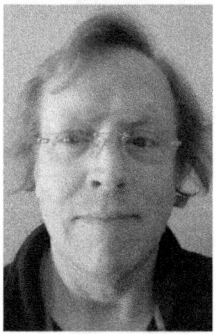

Kenneth C. Dyer, Jr. is a *Healing Minister* and holds an honorary *Doctor of Metaphysics* degree from the *Universal Life Church* based upon life experience and self-study. He's been practicing the Japanese energy healing art of *Reiki* since 1997 and has been a *Master Teacher* since 2007. This healing art opened the door to his study of other areas including Medical Intuition, Aromatherapy, Reflexology, Hypnotism, Herbalism and Nutritional Medicine. He's also a former CNA (*Certified Nurse's Assistant*) and has a Certification in *Herbal Medicine* from the *Herbal Healer Academy.*

Immersed in self-study on numerous topics for many years, and an avid book reader, he researches topics that include holistic healing and natural medicine, psychic phenomenon, the theory of evolution and ID (intelligent design), UFO's and extraterrestrial life, religion and mythology, spirituality and quantum physics, politics and so-called "conspiracy theories", alternative power and off the grid "survivalist" techniques, among many other topics.

Ken has no religious beliefs and rejects organized religion and all forms of unthinking, faith based dogma, but he's a very spiritual person. He knows that in this day and age science and spirituality are merging and each one compliments the other. He also knows that today's religion is tomorrow's mythology. He doesn't like to label himself, but as a very spiritual person he embraces eastern mysticism and philosophy such as Taoism, Confucianism and Buddhism. He finds the idea of a holographic universe utterly fascinating, and considers those things to have many answers to various metaphysical questions. When asked "What religion are you?" he always answers "I am spiritual but not religious". When asked "Do you believe in God?" he typically replies "Not the traditional God, but I do believe in a 'higher power'". His favorite spiritual text is the *Tao Te Ching* from ancient China and he loves reading the books of the Indian mystic OSHO.

A music lover (rock and roll in particular) and musician from childhood, Ken also plays guitar and bass and has current ambitions to form an alternative/hard rock band with himself on bass.

He is the author of two other book titles including *LOVE - EVOLVE - TRANSCEND: Building a Spiritual Culture on the Planet Earth* and *Praise the Lord and Pass the Ammunition.* His website *LoveEvolveTranscend.com.*

Kenneth C. Dyer, Jr.

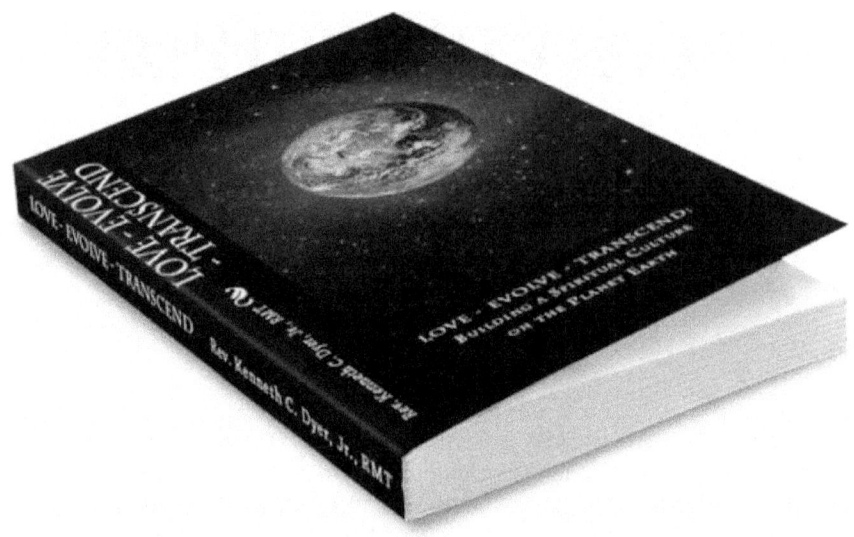

"LOVE - EVOLVE - TRANSCEND: BUILDING A SPIRITUAL CULTURE ON THE PLANET EARTH"

B&W Paperback Edition

or

Deluxe FULL COLOR E-Book Edition (.pdf format)

Available at:

www.loveevolvetranscend.com

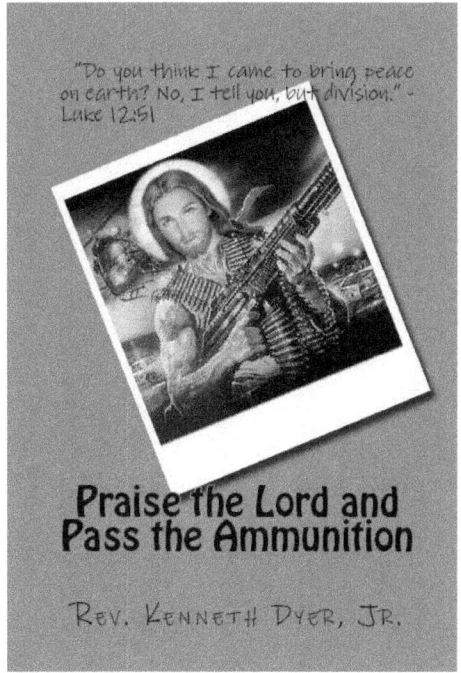

"PRAISE THE LORD AND PASS THE AMMUNITION"

B&W Paperback Edition

or

Deluxe FULL COLOR E-Book Edition
(.pdf format)

Available at:

www.loveevolvetranscend.com

www.ingramcontent.com/pod-product-compliance
Lightning Source LLC
Chambersburg PA
CBHW051859170526
45168CB00001B/170